Irritable Bowel Syndrome

A Practical Guide

GEOFF WATTS

Irritable
Bowel Syndrome

A Practical Guide

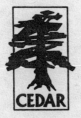

A Mandarin Paperback

IRRITABLE BOWEL SYNDROME: A PRACTICAL GUIDE

First published in Great Britain 1990 by Cedar
an imprint of Mandarin Paperbacks
Michelin House, 81 Fulham Road, London SW3 6RB

Mandarin is an imprint of the Octopus Publishing Group

Copyright © 1990 by Geoff Watts

A CIP catalogue record for this book
is available from the British Library
ISBN 0 434 11170 8

Printed in Great Britain
by Cox & Wyman Ltd, Reading

To D.E.

Acknowledgements

My thanks to June Hall
and Lucinda Culpin
of June Hall Literary Agency,
to Margot Richardson of Mandarin,
to the patients who gave up their time
to talk to me – and likewise the doctors,
especially Professor David Wingate
of the London Hospital.

Contents

Introduction

How are you today? How's your tongue?
Is it smooth and red, or knobbly and
beige with an overcoat of a muddy hue?
And how's the stomach? Is it firm and
steady – or somewhat warm, or a little
wobbly and a trifle windy?

Charles Hill, the Radio Doctor,
speaking on Boxing Day, 1943

There are two things which everyone who suffers from the irritable bowel syndrome should always remember. The first is that no one has ever died of it. It can cause discomfort, distress, and even despair – but not death. To whatever state of misery it reduces sufferers, they do at least have the consolation of knowing that although their illness is a profound nuisance, it is not a medical disaster. The second thing to remember is that some people with the irritable bowel syndrome (IBS for short) find relief through relatively simple measures. No one should allow this wretched disorder to spoil his or her life without at least putting up a fight.

It's impossible to say for certain how many people suffer from the syndrome. The one sure thing is that there are a great many of them. Unfortunately, its victims can't always find the mutual sympathy and support available to people with disorders in which the symptoms are more visible, and of the kind which can be more openly discussed. Severe hay fever, to take one example, can also reduce people to a state of acute misery. But others can see and sympathize with the condition; and talking about it over the dinner table won't upset the hostess or frighten the horses. Even the name 'irritable bowel syndrome' doesn't help. Like tennis elbow, housemaid's knee, and other such disorders with peculiar, improbable, or simply down-to-earth names, a first hearing of the phrase 'irritable bowel syndrome' is more likely to provoke laughter than tears. Sympathy, if it comes, is apt to be an afterthought.

Knowledge, in this century, is power. As far as medicine and health care are concerned, the patients who get the most out of the medical service and their own doctors are those who understand most about their diseases. If you know nothing at all about your disorder, how can you tell if the doctor has tried everything that can be tried? Doctors can't know all there is to be known about every disease. You don't have to tell them how to do their job; indeed, you'd be ill-advised to do any such thing. But well-informed patients can make life easier for doctors by, for example, asking more pertinent questions. A few doctors still prefer to keep their patients in ignorance; but they're a vanishing species.

Of course, it's not strictly necessary to understand anything about an illness you're suffering from; some people are happy to follow the instructions they've been given about how to look after themselves, and prefer to know as little as possible. Personally, I find it easier to do what doctors suggest – and to go on doing so even when I might not feel like it – if I understand the reasons for it all. That's why this book includes not only information about the IBS itself, but also something of what the researchers have found out about the structure of the normal gut, and the way it works in health and in disease. When it comes to treatment, I've also tried to include an outline of the evidence which has led doctors to favour whatever it is they they're prescribing. As often as not, the evidence to support this or that theory about the cause of the IBS, or treatment for it, turns out to be slender. Where this is the case, I see no harm in saying so. My intention is not to undermine patients' hopes, but to inject some sense of realism into their judgements of what can and cannot be done. Given the still limited state of understanding of the irritable bowel syndrome, every attempt to treat it is, in a sense, a partnership in exploration between the doctor and the patient. Such partnerships are best conducted by people who know the true score.

I've also included something about the nature of orthodox and alternative medicine in general. Although this has no unique relevance to the irritable bowel syndrome – what I say would apply just as much to any other disorder – it should help to explain the broad approaches to health and disease taken by the various practitioners whom IBS patients may encounter. The patient who has an insight into their perspectives will have a better idea of what is being suggested, and why.

What this book is not meant to be is a substitute for professional help. No book, however detailed, can take the place of a skilled and knowledgeable human being. However, it is true to say that not all those who advise IBS patients will necessarily have a great deal of knowledge about the disorder. And many who do have the knowledge will be short of time. A book can fill in some of the gaps – or prompt the questions which some patients, in the moment of the consultation, will have forgotten to ask.

I became interested in the irritable bowel syndrome through the weekly BBC programme *Medicine Now* which I present on BBC Radio 4. The first time we broadcast an item on the IBS – I think it was during 1982 – it didn't strike me as much more than a curiosity. At that time I had no idea how many people suffer from the disorder.

What made me realize that it was both common and, perhaps more to the point, not taken entirely seriously by some doctors was the wholly unexpected pile of listeners' letters it provoked. Many of those who had written were clearly delighted just to hear the disorder being discussed on the radio; they found it comforting to be reminded that other people suffer from the IBS, and to know that someone was taking it seriously.

Since that time, the *Medicine Now* office has come to expect a larger than usual postbag whenever the subject crops up. It's one of five topics which have prompted a similar response – and, I suspect, for similar reasons. The others are chronic pain, nausea in pregnancy, myalgic encephalomyelitis (also known as ME, or the post-viral fatigue syndrome) and seasonal affective disorder or winter blues – the last of these being the most recent addition to the list.

In each case the symptoms are vague, and often without much in the way of physical manifestations which would 'prove' that patients are not 'imagining' them. For chronic pain there are all sorts of treatments: the usual indication that no one treatment is strikingly better than all the others, and good for all comers. For the other disorders there are few or even no specific treatments at all. This, of course, is not the fault of the doctors. Where some of them are to blame – and this I've come to gather from reading between the lines of some of the IBS letters I've received – is in showing too little sympathy for patients.

I hope this book will do several things. First, and most obviously, it should answer some of the questions which sufferers want to raise about their illness. Second, I hope it will boost their interest in IBS as a disease. It *is* interesting. Third, it should give the reader some insight into the strengths and the limitations of medicine, and also the way that medical research is carried out. Rather than merely describe what doctors believe about the IBS, I've tried to explain something of the experimental evidence and the reasoning which have led them to these beliefs. And where it's all speculation, I've pointed that out too. Medicine is full of obscure terminology. Where possible, I have tried to avoid it. Where the word has to be used you'll find it in a glossary at the back.

Finally – and perhaps most importantly – I hope this book will offer encouragement to those patients who fear they will have to go on enduring their symptoms indefinitely. This may not be so. New ideas keep on emerging – and with new ideas come the insights which offer researchers new ways of tackling the disease. So take heart, and don't give up hope.

1 The Normal Gut

Harry Secombe: 'Gad, Bloodnok, I admire
your guts.'
Bloodnok: 'What, are they showing?'

From *The Goon Show*, BBC Radio

There are some parts of the human body which seem destined to remain forever on the backburner of our familiarity. How many of us can point exactly and with confidence to the thymus? Or the adrenal glands? Or the spleen? And even if we know roughly where they are, how many of us can say precisely what they do?

There are no such obstacles to hinder our understanding of the gastrointestinal system: the oesophagus, the stomach, the intestines, and their associated openings and exits. We all know where the system starts, and where it ends, and what goes on between. Into the upper end goes food; from the lower end emerge various waste materials; and in between occur the chemical processes which render the one into the other while useful nutrients are first liberated, and then absorbed. All very straightforward. None of the complexity associated with the kidneys or the brain, let alone with the multiplicity of cell types which go to make up the body's immune defence system.

All this is true – and yet to put it so is not to do the gastrointestinal system justice. It isn't quite as straightforward as it seems. Its controls are more sophisticated than they appear. Only in recent years have scientists begun to understand some of the finer points of gut physiology, and to develop a new respect for it as a consequence.

Once food has entered our mouths, we're inclined to think of it as being inside our bodies. In truth it's not – and that becomes clear when you recall how the simplest forms of life absorb their food. A tiny unicellular creature like *Amoeba* – a blob of jelly-like protoplasm which can be found living in most clean pond water, if you've got the microscope to see it – engulfs the nutrients it needs at any convenient point on its outer surface. It's as if you or I put our Sunday lunch through the liquidizer, dropped it into the bath, and then fed ourselves by soaking for an hour or two in the resulting slurry of food.

There's nothing wrong in principle with *Amoeba's* method of feeding. Indeed, because it's so simple, there's a lot to be said in its favour. But as animals become larger, the area of their outer surfaces doesn't increase in proportion to their bulk. Above a certain size there simply isn't enough surface available for this feeding method to be able to cope. An inward extension of the outer surface in the form of a tube running through the body increases the area available for absorbing nutrients. And making that tube longer by curling it upon itself is an obvious means of further boosting its capacity. Moreover the closed environment of the tube allows the organism to bathe relatively large morsels of food in certain chemicals it produces – called enzymes – which reduce them to a more manageable size and, eventually, to a liquid suspension of tiny particles. These enzymes also break down the larger molecules into smaller ones which can be absorbed through the lining of the gut, and into the bloodstream.

Although the human gut is upwards of six metres

(twenty feet) from end to end, this still doesn't provide a surface area large enough to absorb all the nutrients we require. The shortfall is overcome by the ingenious construction of the cells lining the small intestine, the section which forms the greater part of the length of the gut. Its surface isn't smooth, but covered with a vast number of closely packed, tiny, finger-like projections called villi. These boost the effective surface area of the bowel to a level at which it can undertake all the absorption required of it.

The difference between *Amoeba* and ourselves is, then, not quite so great as it might appear. All we have done is to internalize a part of our outer surface. Which is why, even when food has passed through our mouths and down into our stomachs and beyond, it's still 'outside' the body.

Which parts do what

Each section of the tube from mouth to anus has a distinct function. The initial breakdown of food in the mouth is primarily a mechanical affair. But it does have a chemical element to it; chewing promotes the release of saliva which not only lubricates the food for the next stage of its journey, but contains an enzyme called ptyalin. This breaks the large molecules of starch into simpler sugars. So even as the food slips from the mouth into the gullet – the oesophagus – one form of digestion is already underway.

The oesophagus is a little over twenty centimetres (eight inches) long, and its sole function is to convey food from the mouth, through the chest cavity, to the stomach. Its walls are very muscular; when no food is being eaten, they constrict the space between them to almost nothing, effectively closing the tube. As soon as any food enters the upper end of the oesophagus, it is squeezed towards the stomach by a muscular process called peristalsis.

Chewed-up bacon, bananas and biscuits don't drop under gravity from the back of the mouth towards the

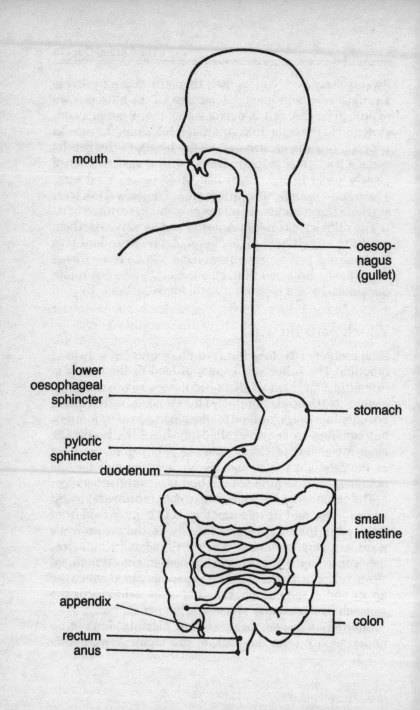

mouth

oesophagus (gullet)

lower oesophageal sphincter

stomach

pyloric sphincter

duodenum

small intestine

appendix

colon

rectum

anus

stomach. Indeed, because of peristalsis, it's possible to swallow while hanging upside down. Peristalsis isn't confined to the gullet; it's found throughout the digestive system. This has to be so because the intestines, squashed into the limited space of the abdominal cavity, are wound upon themselves. The gut contents spend almost as much time moving upwards as they do downwards on their circuitous journey toward the anus. Without peristalsis the pipework would rapidly clog.

The driving force of peristalsis comes from waves of muscular contraction which pass along the length of the oesophagus. Like the rest of the gut, this has two sets of muscles built into its wall. One set runs along the length of the oesophagus; when these longitudinal muscles contract, the region in which they're active becomes shorter and fatter: more bunched up, in other words.

A second set of muscles encircles the oesophagus. When these tighten up they constrict it. The effect of a wave of contraction passing along the oesophagus is rather like that of putting a tennis ball into the mouth of a stocking, closing it off by clenching your fist around the opening, and then sliding your closed fist towards the toe. The tennis ball is pushed along in front of your hand. This principle operates not only in the oesophagus, but in one form or another throughout the rest of the digestive pipework.

The lower end of the oesophagus empties into the upper end of the stomach. To ensure that food doesn't get pushed back up into the oesophagus, a muscular valve called the lower oesophageal sphincter remains closed except when a lump of food is ready to enter the stomach. It's very important that this arrangement works well because the contents of the stomach are extremely acid. Although its lining is designed to cope with this corrosive liquid, that of the oesophagus is not. If the stomach contents do periodically get squirted back up into the gullet, they can cause inflammation and, eventually, ulcers. The opening and closing of this valve is crucial; indeed, as we'll see, muscular co-ordination is central to the smooth operation of the entire gut.

The stomach too is wrapped around with muscle. The upper end can expand, within limits, to accommodate more food as it arrives. Regular waves of contraction (about three per minute) passing through the stomach muscles help to stir the food, and mix it with enzymes which break down proteins into smaller and more easily absorbable molecules. These waves of activity are initiated by electrical signals originating in a pacemaker. In principle this pacing system is not unlike its more celebrated counterpart within the heart.

Just as entry to the upper end of the stomach is controlled by a muscular valve, so too is the exit of food from it. The pyloric sphincter ensures that the partially digested contents of the stomach remain there until they are sufficiently broken down. When the pyloric sphincter opens in response to pressure in the stomach, it does so only enough to allow an outflow of liquid and small particles. In effect, the valve is acting as a sieve.

This valve also prevents a backwash of fluid from the next section of the gut, the duodenum. Much as the oesophagus can be damaged by the stomach contents, so the stomach suffers if the contents of the duodenum are squirted in the wrong direction.

The duodenum itself is about twenty-five centimetres (ten inches) long. The gallbladder and the pancreatic duct carrying a cocktail of digestive enzymes both empty into this section of the small bowel.

On to the small bowel

During the passage of the food through the rest of the small bowel, digestion is completed, and the absorption of nutrients across the gut wall can begin. The six metres (about twenty feet) of the small bowel are coiled up and loosely slung from the back of the abdominal cavity by a tough membrane called the mesentery. This also carries the rich blood supply needed to carry absorbed foods away from the gut.

To allow time for digestion to take place, and for much of the water in the gut to be reabsorbed into the body, the semi-liquid food mustn't be hurried through the small intestine. If the amount of fluid reaching the final section of the gut, the large bowel, exceeds its capacity to absorb water, the result will be diarrhoea. The contents of the small intestine do, though, have to be churned up to ensure that the enzymes responsible for breaking them down are thoroughly mixed in. Freshly digested material also has to be brought into contact with the lining of the gut so that the villi can absorb the liberated nutrients. It follows that the small intestine has to have a rather complicated cycle of contractions which do more than merely move its contents onward.

For this reason the circular muscles of the gut wall make what are known as 'segmentation movements'. Sections of the gut, each an inch or so long, begin to constrict at a rate of up to fifteen squeezes per minute. These sections will then go into a quieter phase of less frequent movement, and other sections of the bowel will adopt this pattern of activity. The overall effect is such as to move the bowel contents onward – but not too fast, at an irregular pace, and sometimes for short distances in the 'wrong' direction.

The final section of the bowel, the large intestine, is something over a metre (about four to five feet) long. The greater part of its length is a tube called the colon. This is much fatter than the small intestine, but otherwise has basically the same structure. By the time the semi-liquid contents of the small intestine have entered the large bowel, most of their nutrients will have been absorbed. This section of the gut is primarily concerned with removing the remaining salt and water – and then thrusting the residue out of the body. Extracting salt and water from the faeces is vital because of the sheer quantity of both which would otherwise be lost. It has been calculated that as much as a gallon and a half of water, and an ounce and a half of salt, are turned over every day by the intestines. These amounts represent about a quarter of the body's total content of both materials. The consequences of a failure to retain them are seen most dramatically in the diarrhoea caused by cholera. Even an adult can die of dehydration in a couple of days if no effort is made to replace the lost salt and water.

Like the small intestine, the large bowel has the type of movement known as segmentation which is designed to churn and squeeze the food residues – in this case to ensure that the water they contain is extracted. Its other movements serve to push the residues along. They take the form of powerful waves of contraction which pass along one section of the bowel. As one wave dies away, another forms itself. When the now firm contents reach the end of the bowel, they're propelled into the rectum. This is about twelve centimetres (five inches) long, and can accommodate 150 grams (four to six ounces) of material. As it fills up with faeces it becomes progressively more distended. This triggers the urge to defecate. The final portion of the gut has more muscular sphincters which keep the bowel firmly shut except when faeces are actually being forced through the anus.

Onwards and outwards

What constitutes a 'normal' bowel habit is matter of dispute and sometimes of passionate debate. Most of what's known about our visits to the lavatory comes from surveys – which, because they rely on subjects' memories, aren't necessarily reliable. With that caveat, more than one study has found that most healthy individuals have between three bowel movements a day, and three a week. This is a fairly wide range – but perhaps no less than might be expected given the variety of our diets, and the differences in determination with which people visit the loo. For what it's worth, the 'average' Western stool weighs about one hundred grams (four ounces). The comparable figure for a Ugandan villager might be as much as four hundred grams.

Transit time – the period separating entry at one end of the gut from exit at the other – has fascinated both the profession and the laity for a century or more. All manner of markers from dyes to radioactive isotopes have been used to measure transit time. One of the more careful studies came up with a figure of two to three days. But the addition of just an ounce of bran reduced the transit time to a day and half. Clearly there's a delicate balance operating here.

Even for clinicians with a total commitment to measuring everything which can be measured, producing averages regarding the consistency of stools and the effort required to pass them represents a mighty challenge. In connection with the former, a substantial minority of people apparently claim that they have to strain at stool – but this is a wholly subjective estimate. One person's Everest is another's Sunday stroll.

Unbelievable though it may seem, one intrepid research group actually devised an instrument for assessing stool consistency. The contraption comprised a small inverted cone which had to be dropped from a standard height on to the newly formed stool. The softer the stool, the greater the depth of penetration – from which its inventors coined a name for their new science: penetrometry.

The point of making or even contemplating measurements like these, except for research purposes, is far from clear. Given that normal healthy people show so much variation, to define a 'normal' bowel habit is about as meaningful as trying to define a 'normal' height. Some people are tall, some are short – and only at the far extremes of stature do we even think of using the word 'abnormal'. Perhaps normality in the question of bowel habit is best thought of as being, within limits, whatever you find most comfortable.

The rhythm of the movements

Returning to the muscular contractions which create all this activity within the gut, their frequency too varies a lot. Most obviously it depends on how much work the gut has to do, which in turn depends on how much food has been eaten. Underlying this variability is a basic rhythm of contractions: a cycle of activity specific to each region of the gut. In the small intestine it's called, rather grandly, the 'migrating motor complex' or MMC. This is a sequence of contractions which starts at the stomach and sweeps through the rest of the gut in the direction of the anus. In the first phase of the cycle, the gut remains inactive for between thirty and sixty minutes. The second phase is one of weak, irregular movements. Finally come five minutes of more powerful contractions – easily perceived, and commonly referred to as hunger pains. The whole MMC cycle starts some three or four hours after completion of a meal, lasts up to two hours, and keeps repeating itself until another meal is eaten.

Two things about gut activity are clear even from this brief description. First, that gut motility is rather more complicated than one might have imagined from simply knowing that undigested food enters at one end, and digested residues are expelled at the other. Second, that to keep all these sets of contractions proceeding smoothly and harmoniously, and to have the various sphincters open and close at the appropriate times, requires a considerable amount of co-ordination. The consequences of peristalsis

going into reverse throughout the whole length of the gut
are too awful to contemplate. Hormones contribute to the
regulation of gut activity; but the major role is played by the
gut's nervous system: another unconsidered trifle which
turns out to be really rather remarkable.

The nerves of the gut

The make up of the body's nervous system – the wiring,
if you like, of our message-carrying and control system –
is complicated and confusing. But unlike the unfortunate
medical student who has to memorize the lot, we need be
concerned only with its broad outlines.

At the heart of the system are the brain and spinal cord –
which together form the central nervous system. The brain,
of course, is ultimately responsible for a great deal of what
happens within our bodies. The variety of its roles is vast.
The lower and evolutionarily more primitive parts concern
themselves with breathing, blood circulation and other
such life-supporting matters which don't require conscious thought or action. They receive information about
the state of the body and its needs, and respond by adjust-
ing these processes to meet those needs. Run up stairs and
signals from the brain will ensure, without you having to
will it, that your heart and lungs both work more rapidly.
The higher centres of the brain are home to our intelli-
gence, our reasoning capacity, and most of the rest of what
makes our species so distinctly different from all others.

The spinal cord is really a downward continuation of
the brain. Its nerves convey messages about the body to
the brain, and carry instructions back. But it's more than
a passive carrier of information. Many reflex responses are
handled by the spinal cord without the need to involve the
brain at all.

Much less well known than the central nervous system
is its second major component, the autonomic nervous

system. This complex of nerves controls many of our bodily functions including reproduction, excretion and digestion. It operates without our conscious control.

Any well-designed control system has to be able to regulate the speed or frequency or intensity or other such characteristics of whatever it's supposed to regulate. The autonomic nervous system achieves this through being split into two branches: they are known as the sympathetic and parasympathetic, and they have opposing influences. Each of the organs they control has a double set of nerves, one from each branch. Nerve impulses arriving along one set encourage the organ to work harder, faster, more often or whatever it may be. Impulses arriving via the other branch have the opposite effect. What actually happens depends on which of the two branches is most active. You can think of it as an interplay between the accelerator pedal and the brake.

In recent years it's become clear that most of the work of regulating the activity of the gut is organized not by the brain, but locally: within the gut itself. Sandwiched between the several layers of the intestinal wall lie two networks of nerve cells. Together they're known as the enteric nervous system. They are found throughout the length of the gut, and they comprise no fewer than five million individual nerve cells. As an indication of the importance of this system in controlling the activity of the bowel, some researchers like to refer to the enteric nervous system as the 'brain in the gut'. These networks do not, of course, operate in isolation; they have many close links with the nerves running into the gut from the brain and spinal cord.

How it all works

Most of the movements of the gut are initiated and co-ordinated by its own nerves: the enteric nervous system. Indeed, if you were to remove the gut from the body and keep it supplied with oxygen and nutrients, it would go on behaving much as it does in the body between meals, with regular cycles of contraction and relaxation. What the 'brain in the gut' can't, of course, be expected to do is regulate gut activity in relation to the wider needs and priorities of the body. If you're attacked and have to run for your life, the last thing your body should be concerned with is digestion. That can wait until the danger has passed. So these duties need to be put temporarily on hold, or at least switched into a lower gear, so that the blood which would otherwise be carrying away absorbed nutrients is available for use by the muscles. It's the autonomic nervous system which is responsible for this regulatory role.

Messages arriving through the sympathetic system generally have an inhibitory effect on gut activity. Messages arriving via the parasympathetic system have the reverse influence: they increase the activity of the gut, and encourage it to secrete more of the enzymes and other materials required for the digestion of food.

Of the two systems, it's the parasympathetic which seems to have the greater day-by-day influence. Cutting the sympathetic nerve supply doesn't have a great deal of effect; indeed, it may be only in emergencies that its inhibitory influence is brought to bear with any great force. Cutting the parasympathetic, on the other hand, results in an immediate shutting down of gut activity – the inference being that under normal circumstances the gut requires a constant prodding to keep up its good work.

To generate even the simplest peristaltic movement is a feat of nervous co-ordination. Each muscle fibre has to be triggered by its nerve supply into contracting at just the right moment, and for the correct length of time. If this doesn't happen, the smooth wave of contraction will degenerate into haphazard twitchings, and the combined power of the tens of thousands of muscle fibres required to force food through the intestine will be lost.

You might compare the role of the enteric nervous system to the computerized switchboard controlling the stage lights in a theatre. For one scene of a play, the lighting director might want a hundred lights, each set to a predetermined brightness. He'll adjust them to achieve exactly the effect he wants, during rehearsal – and then programme the switchboard computer accordingly, instructing it to remember that particular combination. For the next scene he'll readjust everything to give him the new effect he's looking for – and so on. Later, during the performance itself, he can call up whatever pattern of lighting he's chosen for a scene, no matter how complicated it might be, by pressing a single button. In broad terms, this is something like the relationship of the brain to the gut. The brain isn't issuing a complex string of instructions which tell the gut how to form the sequence of muscular contractions required to push its contents along. Rather what it does is issue an instruction to the gut to follow this or that pre-set programme of behaviour – the details of the programme being already stored locally in the wiring of the enteric nervous system.

At least three programmes are available to this system. First there's the pattern of activity it shows between meals: the migrating motor complex. Then there's a pattern of contractions which is stimulated by food. And finally there's a programme for emergency use only; this is the activity required for vomiting if something noxious gets into the system, and has to be expelled.

As researchers study the fine detail of the physiology of the gut, and begin to understand how it works, the picture gets evermore complicated. This may be cold comfort to people suffering from the irritable bowel syndrome – but, as so often with the human body, the more you comprehend the gastrointestinal system, the more you come to marvel that it doesn't fail more often.

2 A Picture of the Syndrome

One finger in the throat and one in the
rectum make a good diagnostician

Sir William Osler

The irritable bowel syndrome may not have a name calculated to win the sympathy of people who've never
suffered from or previously heard of it; but the word
'irritable' is at least apt. It captures something of the
quality of the mixed and often ill-defined collection of
symptoms which make up the syndrome. It suggests a gut
which is sensitive, touchy, and easily provoked. Equally,
it conveys something of one of the consequences for the
sufferer. 'Angry bowel syndrome' would sound altogether
too threatening; the IBS is not in itself a danger to physical
health, or a harbinger of future and more serious disease.
It's a profound nuisance: a source of . . . irritation. *Roget's
Thesaurus* offers half a column of alternatives – none of
which seems quite as appropriate as 'irritable'.

The predominant symptoms of the syndrome are intermittent bouts of pain in the abdomen together with
diarrhoea, or constipation, or alternating diarrhoea *and*
constipation. The diarrhoea may take the form of stools

which are looser than normal, or which need to be passed frequently, or which catch the sufferer with a sudden and unpredictable desire to go to the lavatory. Constipation may mean less frequent visits to the lavatory, the need to strain excessively, or the passage of faeces which are compressed and hard and sometimes bear more resemblance to rabbit droppings than to anything of human origin.

The quality of the pain varies from patient to patient. Pain can be very difficult to describe. While the pain associated with the IBS is usually said to be dull and aching, it may sometimes be sharp and stabbing. It may become so severe as to disrupt daily life – although this is uncommon. Going to the lavatory often relieves it – temporarily, at least. Patients who can localize their pain often feel it in the middle or lower part of the abdomen. Other symptoms which often but not invariably accompany these core features are mucus in the stools, feelings of bloatedness, nausea, vomiting, dyspepsia (indigestion), and excessive stomach rumbling and gurgling. (The technical term for this is 'borborygmus' – which does sound more impressive than 'stomach rumbling'.)

These symptoms may be continuous, but they are more often intermittent. Sometimes they start for no obvious reason. On other occasions their appearance seems to be provoked by a meal, a particular type of food, or some stressful event.

One of the first and most careful studies of patients suffering from the IBS dates from 1962. Drs Nazir Chaudhary and S. C. Truelove of Oxford's Radcliffe Infirmary followed the progress of 130 of their patients for up to three years from the time of diagnosis. Their group included twice as many women as men; most of the women were aged between twenty and sixty, and many of the men were in their forties. IBS symptoms aside, most of them were in good physical health. A quarter had been suffering from their illness for more than ten years, and nearly all had had it for some considerable time. More than a third claimed that their symptoms were exacerbated if they ate certain foods: notably fruit (especially apples, pears and oranges), tomatoes, fresh salads and anything fried. About a quarter thought that the onset of their symptoms had followed a gut infection of some kind. Most complained of a sense of fatigue, a loss of concentration, and depression or anxiety. In special interviews devoted to psychological aspects of the disorder, Dr Chaudhary and his colleague subsequently confirmed the existence of these and other such psychological factors. Some of the matters which they felt to be important included marital difficulties, anxiety over children or parents, sexual difficulties, business and financial worries, and a fear of cancer.

With treatment, nearly all the IBS patients showed at least some improvement. Those in whom psychological factors seemed to be playing a part tended to do less well.

The entire gut – or just part of it?

By and large, the irritable bowel syndrome is thought of as a disorder of the large intestine. However, many patients also complain of symptoms which seem more likely to have arisen from other regions of the gastrointestinal tract: these symptoms include heartburn, nausea and belching. There's also a certain amount of experimental evidence which points in the same direction. IBS patients have been shown to have disturbances of the normal pattern of contraction of the oesophagus, and of the small bowel. A few years ago, Professor Nicholas Read of the Royal Hallamshire Hospital in Sheffield studied the passage of food through the guts of patients with the IBS, and through those of normal healthy control subjects. After an overnight fast, each one ate a standard meal comprising sausages, baked beans and mashed potato followed by pineapple and custard. (You can tell this research was being conducted in a British NHS hospital.) The researchers used two methods of following the food on its journey: a radioactive isotope and a known number of small pieces of plastic tube which were radio-opaque, and would therefore show up on X-ray pictures. Both isotope and plastic tubes were hidden in the mashed potato.

When the subjects had finished their meals, each was asked to lie down, and to remain in that position for at least six hours. In the meantime, the researchers measured the rate at which the food left each subject's stomach by recording the amount of radioactivity within it at various times after the beginning of the experiment. To find out how long the first of the stomach contents took to pass the length of the small intestine and reach the beginning of the large bowel they used the hydrogen breath test (for details, see page 74). By taking X-ray pictures of each subject's stools, and then counting the number of pieces of plastic which had emerged from the body, the researchers were able to deduce the transit time for the whole gut. (Ingenuity is one of the hallmarks of gastrointestinal science.)

The data suggest that different patterns of symptoms in the IBS, such as constipation and diarrhoea, are related to differing transit times through the small bowel – though how isn't entirely clear. Although the time taken for food to get through the small bowel did not differ significantly between patients and healthy control subjects, it may be that the colon of IBS patients is less able to tolerate the variations in small bowel transit time that are found even in normal guts. There is evidence (acquired by inflating small balloons inside the guts of conscious subjects and asking them what they feel) that IBS patients are unduly sensitive to distention of the gut wall. Professor Read's research revealed a marked correlation between the time at which the test meals entered the patients' colons, and the time at which those individuals began to complain of abdominal pain. Exactly how the small bowel might be involved in generating the symptoms of the IBS is still obscure; but it does seem to have a role of some kind. We'll return to it later in Chapter 10.

Defining the IBS

When you consider that virtually all of us can expect to suffer one or more of the symptoms of the IBS from time to time, it's clear why doctors have had some difficulty in framing a satisfactory definition of the syndrome. The further difficulty is that the IBS is what doctors describe as a 'functional' disorder. At first hearing this phrase is rather peculiar. People whose kidneys have failed are suffering from a kidney malfunction; people with severe head injuries have a loss of brain function, and so on. Indeed, most of medicine is about a loss of function in this or that organ or system of the body. In fact, doctors use the term 'functional disorder' to disguise what is really an admission of ignorance. It's applied to those disorders in which the root cause is unknown, and the only apparent abnormality is the malfunction itself. The cause of the lost brain function following a severe head injury are all too apparent. But there's nothing like this in the case of the IBS. The patients suffering from IBS symptoms are in most respects indistinguishable from those without them. The disorder can only be defined in terms of the changes in bowel function – and as this is enormously variable, the definition of the disease inevitably becomes rather arbitrary. Of course, there must be something which underlies the IBS, and sets off the symptoms which the patient then recognizes. This 'something', this fundamental cause, is what the researchers are now trying to find – and I'll be discussing current thinking about what it might be in later chapters.

In desperation, some definitions of the irritable bowel

syndrome have been based on the exclusion principle: in other words, the irritable bowel syndrome is what's left over when examinations and tests have ruled out everything else. This is hardly ideal. So, in 1988, a working party commissioned by the International Congress of Gastroenterology grasped the nettle and came up with the following definition:

A functional gastrointestinal disorder attributable to the intestines with:
○ abdominal pain;
○ symptoms of disturbed defecation (urgency, straining, feelings of incomplete evacuation, altered stool form or consistency, and altered bowel frequency/timing);
○ bloatedness (distension).

It's conceivable that what we refer to as the irritable bowel syndrome is actually more than one disorder. Some doctors therefore prefer to split the syndrome into sub-groups depending on the patient's symptoms. The commonest division is into just two categories. Many patients fall into the group who have pain plus constipation which sometimes alternates with diarrhoea. In the second division are patients mainly troubled by diarrhoea without much pain, often at its worst in the morning.

An alternative is to split the IBS into no fewer than five categories. First there are patients with a spastic colon. (This is actually one of the older terms for what is now called the IBS.) Individuals in this category are those whose abdominal pain is relieved by going to the lavatory, who experience altered frequency and consistency of bowel movements, and who suffer feelings of abdominal distension and incomplete evacuation after defecation. In the second category are patients who suffer from painless diarrhoea. This would be defined as passing loose, runny stools during more than a quarter of visits to the lavatory. Next there is 'atonic constipation' in which the rectum is usually full, the patient may have less than three bowel movements a week, and strains to pass stools on more than a quarter of all occasions. Fourthly there are patients whose predominant problem is gas: a problem usually improved by starvation and eased by flatulence. Finally there is a group of patients who have suffered from abdominal pain on three or more days a week for more than a year. This pain is usually unrelated to meals or bowel habit.

You may think that all this categorization is rather pointless: the mere gratification of an urge to have everything neatly packaged and labelled. To be honest, there are some doctors too who would take that view. But definitions in medicine *are* important for reasons other than mere tidy-mindedness. Research involving patients becomes virtually useless if different groups of doctors can't agree on exactly what was wrong with a particular group of patients for whom a new treatment worked well. To take an extreme example, diarrhoea is a feature of cholera, and of Salmonella food poisoning. But the doctor who lumped together all such patients on the grounds that all had this particular symptom would be unlikely to discover much about the causes of either disease. His patients wouldn't be particularly grateful either.

Non-gut symptoms

Before going on to consider who is most likely to develop the irritable bowel syndrome, it's worth noting that some sufferers also have an appreciable number of non-gut symptoms. One study carried out in Manchester compared one hundred IBS patients with one hundred healthy people of similar age, sex and social class. The results showed that the IBS patients had a much greater number of symptoms which appeared to have nothing to do with the gut. They had more urinary symptoms (such as frequency and urgency), more gynaecological symptoms (including pre-menstrual tension and painful periods), and more non-specific symptoms (back pain, headaches, tiredness, poor sleeping and so on). They also had more psychological problems – but the issue of gut and brain is one I'll be returning to in more detail.

The same researchers also made a study of women with the irritable bowel syndrome and found that more than eight out of every ten of them had severe pain or other difficulties during sexual intercourse. Of course it might be that all gut complaints create sexual difficulties for women. The researchers checked this by asking the same questions of women with two other intestinal disorders: duodenal ulcers and inflammatory bowel disease. Sexual difficulties turned out to be only a quarter to a third as common in these patients – so there does seem to be a more specific connection with the IBS.

The sufferers

No one knows how many people suffer from the irritable bowel syndrome – but the number is obviously large because it accounts for between two and five out of every ten people referred to hospital gastroenterologists. Interestingly, what has become clear from surveys is that far more people have symptoms of the disorder than actually seek medical help for it. One of the best surveys of this kind was organized jointly by Drs Ken Heaton of the Bristol Royal Infirmary, and Grant Thompson of the Ottawa Civic Hospital in Canada. They questioned several groups of subjects: male medical technicians and female nurses in training; a randomly selected population of people attending a heart disease screening clinic; a number of female hospital clerical staff; and finally the residents of some old people's flats. This gave them three age categories – young, middle-aged and elderly – each with about one hundred subjects. Using detailed questionnaires they tried to find out which of their subjects had any of the symptoms of a functional gut disorder.

Abdominal pain, straining when defecating, urgency, feelings of distension and many of the other symptoms already described were all quite common. More than a tenth of the people interviewed – all, in their own opinion and to the best of their knowledge, healthy – had the symptom pattern typical of the irritable bowel syndrome. But few of them had consulted a doctor. What these figures mean is an issue I'll be considering later. The lesson for the moment is that as far as the IBS is concerned there is, to use the time-honoured phrase, a lot of it about.

Because the IBS is so difficult to define, is so subjective, and has symptoms which are so common, some doctors have wondered if it should really be described as a disease at all. To grasp what they're getting at, consider another quality of human beings: their height. There is no such thing as a 'normal' height. There is an average height, and the further you depart from that average – above it or below it – the fewer the people who have that particular stature. But very little of this variation would be regarded as in any way the manifestation of an illness. Only at the far extremes does the word 'disorder' begin to enter the picture. Gigantism, for example, is an abnormality of growth which is caused by the overproduction during childhood of a hormone called somatotrophin. The more of the hormone you have, the taller you become. Conversely, a child who fails to make enough of the hormone will remain abnormally short. Doctors intervene in both these situations in an effort to correct the hormone level.

Could most cases of the irritable bowel syndrome be nothing more than the fluctuations in functional efficiency which most biological systems exhibit from time to time? After all, few of the body's organ systems can be expected to operate to perfection for seventy or eighty years. Living machines are vastly more reliable than their manmade counterparts; but they do have their limits. There is no obvious answer to this question of whether or not the IBS is a 'real' disease – which is anyway more of a philosophical than a practical issue. The fact is that large numbers of people know that their gastrointestinal systems are causing them considerable distress and annoyance. If this can be understood and remedied, it matters relatively little whether the enterprise is described as 'curing a disordered body process' or 'improving the efficiency of an otherwise normal body process'.

This aside, the patients who do go to a doctor are predominantly in their third to fifth decade of life, fit, female and (in North America) white. Patients diagnosed after the age of thirty-five usually seem to have had a history of bowel disturbance dating from childhood or adolescence. Their misery has been long-lived.

Diagnosis

As already pointed out, defining the irritable bowel syndrome as what's left over when everything else has been ruled out is less than satisfactory. In practice, though, diagnosis still has to be based on more or less that principle. The reasons are simple enough: for one thing there is no test specific for the IBS alone; for another the commonest symptoms of the IBS are also those of a variety of other gut disorders – some of them a good deal more worrisome. Diarrhoea and/or constipation with or without abdominal pain may also be caused by diverticular disease, certain parasitic infections, inflammatory bowel diseases such as ulcerative colitis, bacterial infections (including Salmonella), various tumours, and a number of other things.

The doctor will want to eliminate all these before settling for a diagnosis of the irritable bowel syndrome. It's said that most gastroenterologists soon develop an instinct for identifying IBS patients; but any doctor who relies solely on instinct is doing no service to the patients, and is sooner or later likely to find himself on the sharp end of a negligence action. In the first instance the GP may try to do something about the problem himself. He'll start by asking you for details of all your symptoms, and how long you've had them. He'll want to be sure that they aren't due to the use of excessive amounts of laxatives (the British, in particular, are notorious for our obsessional interest in our bowels, and our desire to alter the frequency of their opening!) or the result of some other drug which is being taken. He may also ask a lot of questions which seem to be irrelevant, but which may help him to carry out that process of elimination already mentioned. Doctors (who like to describe even simple things in peculiar, complicated, or – as in this case – faintly poetic terms) call this 'taking a history'.

Besides asking about physical symptoms, the doctor will also inquire if you have been under stress, either at work or at home, or if you've been feeling depressed. He'll be especially interested in anything which coincided with the onset of the IBS symptoms.

During his initial physical examination he will prod the abdomen, searching for signs of tenderness or rigidity in the superficial muscles, or in the large bowel. But in the nature of gut problems, there's not much to be felt from the outside, and even less to be seen. It's common to do some blood tests, and also to send a stool specimen to the laboratory to check that it doesn't contain any blood invisible to the naked eye. It may also be tested for the presence of bacteria, or some more exotic intruder, especially if you've recently taken a trip to a tropical country. Blood in the stools can point to the presence of a growth

– malignant or otherwise – in the bowel. Even before this stage, the GP may have decided that a specialist opinion is called for. Either way, further investigation is the province of the hospital gastroenterologist – to whom the patient will now be referred.

Hospital investigations

The problem now is to decide what further investigations need to be done. Given the ingenuity of medical researchers, all sorts of things are possible. But what's possible isn't necessarily what's sensible. The caring doctor wants to reassure the patient, not frighten him or her to death with a series of (sometimes) rather unpleasant investigations which go beyond what's required simply to be certain that nothing life-threatening is involved. What the specialist decides to do will depend on the patient's symptoms. If the main one is diarrhoea, the task may be rather more problematic; a slightly greater range of disorders will have to be excluded before the specialist can satisfy himself that the complaint he's dealing with really is functional, and not organic (that is, when a specific chemical or structural abnormality can be traced).

The procedure which pretty well all doctors agree upon is known as sigmoidoscopy. The object is to examine the interior of the large bowel: an intention which must be realized in the obvious manner, and by the only available route. The instrument used to make the examination is called a sigmoidoscope. There's nothing new about peering up into the large bowel. Hippocrates had a go at it, though not until the 1800s did doctors begin using instruments bearing some dim resemblance to those now in use. Today's devices still comprise little more than a rigid viewing tube with a small light source at its tip. The invention of fibre optics – in essence bundles of flexible glass fibres – made possible the development of viewing tubes which can bend, and so be steered around corners while still allowing the operator to see through them. Instruments which thus allow the operator to peer into the further reaches of the large bowel are known as colonoscopes.

The presence of too much material in the large bowel will prevent the easy passage of the viewing tube, and also obscure the operator's view. For this reason the bowel may have to be cleared using an enema. The patient lies on one side, with knees pulled up to his chest. The surgeon may first explore the rectum using a gloved and lubricated finger. Having satisfied himself that there is nothing to prevent the smooth passage of the sigmoidoscope, he will then insert it through the anus – again, well lubricated. No anaesthesia is usually needed, but some patients will be given a sedative. The procedure is not comfortable, but it shouldn't be painful. If it proves to be so, tell the doctor immediately.

The sigmoidoscope incorporates a small pump which allows the doctor to inflate the bowel. This serves two purposes; it helps him to push the instrument on its way; and it also improves his view of the interior of the bowel. What he sees will depend on the type of symptoms suffered by that particular patient. In someone who mainly experiences abdominal pain and constipation (the spastic type of IBS) he may well be able to see the lower end of the bowel contracting violently and repeatedly. This has been described, rather engagingly, as the 'winking sign'. Inflating the colon sometimes causes the very pain of which the patient has been complaining. This can be reassuring because it does indicate that the pain is related simply to the muscular actions of the gut wall, and not to something more sinister.

If sigmoidoscopy reveals nothing out of the ordinary, the doctor will have taken an important step towards diagnosing the irritable bowel syndrome. But other tests ruling out other possibilities may still be needed. The next most likely is a barium enema. This is a way of using X-rays to take a picture of the large bowel. X-rays pass easily through soft tissues, and ordinary X-ray pictures are really only useful for seeing bone. One way of making structures like the gut show up more clearly is to coat their inside with something which is opaque to X-rays. Barium is such a material. For the stomach and upper reaches of the bowel, it's most convenient to put the barium in at the top end. But for the large bowel it makes more sense to use the lower end. Taking the barium by this route is messier and less comfortable – but at least you don't have to swallow the stuff.

Patients having a barium enema may be asked to take a laxative the night before the procedure, and to make sure they open their bowels on the morning of the day itself. The doctor inserts a tube into the rectum, and then uses it to run in a barium-containing fluid. When the required X-ray pictures have been taken, the fluid will be run back out through the tube, or disposed of into the lavatory. The only after-effect may be a certain amount of wind. Examination of the resulting X-ray pictures should show up anything untoward inside the gut.

There are other investigations which the doctor can request if he still isn't certain that an organic cause for the patient's symptoms should be ruled out. But assuming that the laboratory tests reveal nothing abnormal, it's at this stage that he'll most likely make his diagnosis. And having decided that the problem really is the irritable bowel syndrome, he'll begin pondering how best to overcome it.

3 What Makes the Bowel Irritable?

A disease known is half cured.

Proverb

As pointed out in the last chapter, the irritable bowel syndrome is categorized as a 'functional' disorder – which simply means that no one really knows what causes it. Like nature, medical theorists abhor a vacuum; so there's no shortage of suggested causes.

Unless you believe in divine intervention as the cause of each and every bout of illness, all disease has a physical explanation of some kind. It may be a consequence of something you've eaten or drunk or inhaled; it may be due to a microbe which has entered your body; it may be the outcome of exposure to hazardous chemicals; it may relate to something which happened yesterday or last week or twenty years ago; it may be a direct result of age-related changes in your body; or it may stem from stressful or other emotional experiences which, through the brain and nervous system, have led to organic changes in the way your body works. There are numerous plausible explanations. The challenge is to establish which is correct.

There are also many reasons for wanting to know which explanation is correct, but two of them stand out as being most important. First there are the obvious practical considerations; by knowing why something has gone wrong there is a better chance of being able to put it right. Beyond that, though, there's the purely intellectual dimension. Humans have always wanted to know how things work, and why they go wrong. It's a characteristic of our species – and nothing is intrinsically more fascinating than trying to find out how our bodies work. There is, unfortunately, no easy way of seeking these answers. Common sense and intuition may be good starting points, but that's all they are. Watch the sun rise in the morning, travel in its long arc across the sky, then set in the evening, and common sense tells you that the sun must circle the earth. Common sense just happens to be wrong. Any person who says that he 'knows' what causes the irritable bowel syndrome is best treated with scepticism. Ask how he knows; ask what he's done to prove he's right; and then look critically at his proof.

Before going through some of the current theories, it might be helpful to spend a little more time unpicking that term 'functional'. Because it's used to describe diseases of unknown cause, there will come a time (we hope) when each disorder shakes off this label. The case of lactose intolerance provides an example which is directly relevant to the bowel.

Lactose intolerance

Lactose is a type of sugar found in milk. In normal circumstances an enzyme, lactase, produced by the small intestine breaks it down into its smaller constituent molecules. Unlike their parent molecule, these constituents are small enough to be absorbed in the usual way through the gut wall. If the body doesn't make enough lactase, some undigested lactose may pass on into the large intestine. Here bacteria ferment it to produce lactic acid. This causes diarrhoea and feelings of abdominal discomfort: the symptoms of lactose intolerance.

Back in 1975, a Sudanese doctor then working in Edinburgh described in the medical journal *The Lancet* how his life since the age of nine or ten had been profoundly disturbed by a series of bowel disturbances which included pain, rumbling, flatulence and diarrhoea. He recalls how at boarding school he became famous for blocking access to the toilets for hours on end. And the condition created religious problems. 'The frequent passage of flatus,' he wrote, 'imposed a great difficulty in performing prayers, for it invalidates the ritual of washing which is necessary before each of the five-times-daily Moslem prayers.' Although outwardly he tried to make a joke of the whole thing, inwardly he was deeply troubled.

Medical advice, both conventional and from a local healer, proved useless. On entering medical school he diagnosed himself as having cancer – but later decided he was actually suffering from the irritable bowel syndrome. 'I came to believe that my disturbed, introspective, neurotic and obsessional personality must have selected my bowel as its target.'

In 1973 he came to Britain. Here his symptoms became even worse – a change he attributed to the stress of adapting to a new country, and also to examinations:

Daily work became an ordeal. Although I took only a light breakfast of cornflakes and milk, the ward rounds became intolerable. I had to suppress volumes of flatulence and abdominal rumbling and after the rounds I would rush home to the toilet to have several explosive bowel actions.

Having begun work as a gastroenterologist (was this fate, chance, or a conscious quest for self-understanding?) he became even more convinced that his problem was the irritable bowel syndrome. Accordingly he began to eat bran every morning, washed down with . . . yes, milk. But this made things worse. A chance remark to a colleague prompted the suggestion that his problem might not be an irritable bowel, but a case of lactose intolerance. A dose of pure lactose – which provoked a swift homeward departure from the hospital followed by ten hours of raging diarrhoea – confirmed that this was indeed the case:

> Within a few days of starting a milk-free diet, I found that I had lost the persistent abdominal distension and the need to pass flatus so frequently. My abdominal rumbling disappeared and for almost the first time in my life I had regular bowel actions.

This little saga has many lessons. It shows that doctors make bad diagnosticians when confronted with their own symptoms. It shows how people are often inclined to fear the worst (for instance, cancer). It demonstrates how symptoms which are such a source of public merriment can also make life a misery for the sufferer. And, most important, it shows how symptoms as tiresome as those of the irritable bowel can arise from a simple and otherwise inconsequential inability to make a particular enzyme. Of course, once the cause of this doctor's bowel disturbance had been understood it could no longer be described as a functional disorder; it had a straightforward organic cause. The hope is that other irritable bowels will prove to have equally identifiable causes which can be equally easily remedied. If this is so, the catch-all diagnosis 'irritable bowel syndrome' will become progressively rarer, and be replaced by several or perhaps many more exact labels. So far, it has to be admitted, the researchers – and thus the sufferers – haven't had a great deal of success. Functional problems they are, and functional problems they remain, most of these irritable bowels.

Fibre

The simplest of the theories about the irritable bowel syndrome is that it results from eating a diet containing too little fibre. Dietary fibre (or roughage, to use the older and now outmoded term) has undergone a radical change of image in the past decade. An interest in it was once the exclusive province of food faddists and the supporters of various back-to-nature movements. Now it's become not merely respectable, but trendy.

The term 'fibre' is used to describe a mixture of plant materials which resist digestion by the enzymes of the small intestine. Much of it is cellulose, the insoluble material which makes up the walls of plant cells, and which is most familiar to us in the form of cotton and paper. Soluble components of fibre include pectin, the material found in soft fruits, which contributes to the setting of jam. A third ingredient, lignin, is the stuff which gives plant stems their woody quality. Besides these three materials, there are at least three more which collectively constitute fibre. Foods rich in dietary fibre include leafy vegetables, many fruits and, of course, bran. What you get depends on what you eat.

Not all this material passes right through the body; some of its ingredients can be broken down by bacteria living in the large bowel. The extent to which this happens in humans is limited; herbivorous animals like cows, on the other hand, derive a significant part of their nutrients in this way. The variety and chemical composition of fibre is complicated; and this has led to disagreements about how best to define and measure it. Naturally enough this tends to complicate research on its effects.

The history of man's interest in fibre (albeit not by that name) goes back at least to the time of Hippocrates. He noted, with some approval, that wholemeal bread increases the quantity of stools passed. But later authorities were less sympathetic, and fibre in the form of wholemeal bread suffered a loss of favour which lasted for more than two millennia. White was smart when it came to flour, and the whiter the better. Wholemeal flour and bread were foods to be eaten only if you couldn't afford anything else. Not until nutrition had developed as a science did it become clear that bran – the outer covering of the wheat grain – contains useful vitamins and minerals as well as fibre. The 'national loaf', introduced by the British government during World War II and rich in bran, was an economy measure designed to make the most of all available foodstuffs. Its beneficial effects upon constipation were noted; seldom, before or since, have British bowels opened more often or to greater effect. But still fibre continued to be undervalued, not least by doctors.

The restoration of fibre to medical respectability was brought about principally by three men. They were Surgeon Captain T.L. Cleave, author of a book called The Saccharine Disease, and his later supporters the Rev. Dr Hugh Trowell and Dr Dennis Burkitt. The argument put forward in the The Saccharine Disease was that the removal of fibre from the diet, and the increasing amount of refined carbohydrate which tended to replace it are responsible for many of the ills of civilized society: not only obesity, dental caries and cancer of the colon but also – and more controversially – peptic ulcers, gout, high blood pressure and acne. A high fibre diet is, of course, the key element in the extremely successful 'F-plan Diet'. This is not the place to go further into the pros and cons of the fibre theory – about which in any case it's still impossible to reach a final conclusion. Different forms of fibre, for example, have different effects. And there are disagreements about their practical significance. But many of the actions of fibre are now well known and widely accepted.

What fibre does

Fibre retards the absorption of glucose and, to some extent, fat from the intestine and so slows its entry into the bloodstream. It's therefore recommended for diabetes and, with rather less conviction, for people seeking to reduce their blood cholesterol levels. Less encouragingly there has been some concern that too much fibre might prevent the absorption of some necessary minerals from the gut. As far as the gut itself is concerned, a high fibre diet tends to expand, soften and so increase the bulk of the stools. Dr Dennis Burkitt, working in Uganda, noticed that the stools of Africans (he has an eye for these things) could be as much as four times larger than those of the local white population. Observant travellers in the Third World continue to find opportunities (all too many of them) to verify this assertion for themselves. Food also passes through the bodies of Africans up to twice as quickly. It soon became clear that diet was at the root of these differences.

In recent years ideas have changed about the way in which fibre achieves its bulking effect. The less digestible forms of fibre, including coarse bran, create some effect in the obvious manner: simply by being there. But this alone could hardly account for the greatly increased volume of the stools. It was then suggested that what counts is fibre's capacity to increase the amount of water retained in the stools: the greater the amount of water present, the greater the bulk. But this idea too had to be modified when it was realized that some bulking agents disappear almost entirely from the colon, yet still have an effect on the quantity of its contents. It's now thought that some forms of fibre are at least partially digested by bacteria living within the colon; and it's the mass of dead bacteria so formed which accounts for much of the bulking effect. The more voluminous the stools, the more rapidly the muscles of the colon expel them from the body.

The belief that irritable bowels have something to do with a low fibre diet has been prompted by the prevalence of the condition in those (mainly Western) countries which eat food of this type. Doctors who have worked in Africa certainly claim that the irritable bowel is a rarity on that continent – though if there is indeed a link between diet and the IBS, it surely won't be long before urbanized Africans start to share the intestinal burdens of their sometime colonizers. Of course, the fact that a particular remedy helps to overcome a disorder doesn't mean that it was the absence of that remedy which created the problem. A headache may respond to aspirin; but it wasn't the absence of aspirin which triggered the headache.

Why having less solid material in the gut should produce the symptoms of the irritable bowel syndrome is a matter of speculation. It could be argued that the circumstances under which our gastrointestinal system evolved fitted it for dealing with rather more fibre than can be found in a diet of McDonalds hamburgers, ice cream and Coca Cola. Under these circumstances the gut, geared up to propel more solid residues than are actually present, finds itself with nothing on which to press. Whether this alone could be held to account for all the symptoms of the IBS is surely doubtful. Either way, it's also clear that fibre speeds up the transit time of food residues through the gut, and reduces the pressure within the colon.

Perhaps lack of fibre is best thought of as a contributory factor rather than a cause of the IBS in its own right. While each of two people might have whatever abnormality of gut physiology underlies the syndrome, only the one who eats too little fibre would be disturbed by it. The fibre, in this case, would be serving to disguise the underlying disorder. There is some experimental evidence to support this view of the role of fibre. Recordings made of the electrical activity of the muscles of the bowel of people with the IBS are different from those of normal, healthy individuals. And even when treatment with bran has overcome the symptoms, the underlying abnormalities of electrical activity can still be detected.

Food intolerance

A quite different and more controversial theory about the irritable bowel syndrome has been pursued by Dr John Hunter and colleagues at Addenbrooke's Hospital in Cambridge. They've been exploring the possibility that the IBS is caused by food intolerance.

The topic of food intolerance has become enormously confused in recent years. This confusion has arisen partly because it's now very fashionable to claim that all sorts of maladies are the result of adverse reactions to foodstuffs, and partly also through a loose use of terminology. Taking the second point first, 'food intolerance' means an abnormal reaction to a specific food. The symptoms of food intolerance are extremely mixed, but include headache, fatigue, recurrent mouth ulcers, nausea, diarrhoea, constipation and joint pains.

There are many reasons why a person may not be able to tolerate certain foods: one of these reasons may be that he or she has a specific type of food intolerance – called 'food allergy'. This is an adverse reaction to food involving the body's immune defence system. It's a kind of gastronomic equivalent of hay fever; common examples of allergy-provoking foods are eggs, strawberries, nuts and shellfish. There are specific tests by which it's possible to tell if an adverse reaction to a food involves the immune system, and should therefore be categorized as a food allergy.

Unfortunately, some of the gurus who flourish in this field have insisted on referring to all adverse reactions as 'food allergies'. They like to claim that immunologists have hijacked the term and given it a narrower application than was originally intended. Although the dispute is trivial and foolish, it can nonetheless have some tiresome or even damaging consequences. Someone who's read that all adverse reactions to food are properly described as 'food allergies' may go to the doctor claiming that he or she has just such a problem. If the appropriate tests are then performed, but prove negative, the doctor will be entitled to say that that person is not suffering from a food allergy. This is likely to be interpreted as meaning, 'It's all in your mind. Go away and stop bothering me.' All the doctor may have meant to say is, 'It's some other form of food intolerance you've got.' The confusion and distress which can arise out of the failure to untie these semantic knots has to be seen to be believed. Doctors and patients who fully understand what's going on in each other's heads are seldom confused by such an issue. But how many doctors and patients do have such an understanding?

Dr Hunter and his colleagues set up some careful experiments designed to avoid the many pitfalls which bedevil work in this field. Their first study involved twenty-five patients suffering the classic symptoms of the irritable bowel syndrome. All were asked to limit their eating to a single meat, a single fruit, and distilled or spring water, and to continue in this way for a whole week. Four of the patients refused even to try the diet – which is not really surprising when you think how tedious it must be to live like this. Fourteen patients were delighted to find that their symptoms rapidly cleared up. Each was then asked to go on eating the same diet, but reintroducing one extra item of food daily until the IBS symptoms reappeared. The aim was to pin down whichever food (or foods) had been causing the problem. In order of frequency, the following turned out to be the troublemakers: wheat (in bread, cakes, and so on), corn, dairy products, coffee, tea, and citrus fruits.

In their next study, Dr Hunter and colleagues aimed to confirm the results of the previous experiments, and also to trace the roots of this food intolerance. Six of the patients who had become free of all symptoms following the week on the exclusion diet agreed to go into hospital for four days. On each day they ate an identical diet comprising foods which posed no problem for them. Breakfast, though, was a little different – which is putting it mildly. Each subject first had a tube pushed up the nose, down the back of the throat and on into the stomach. A nurse then fed these forbearing individuals 'breakfast' in the form of a liquidized preparation of one particular foodstuff. Each morning the patients received one of two different foods: either something to which they claimed to react badly, or something which was no problem for them. Neither the nurse nor the subject knew which of the two foods were being provided on which days – and because their tastebuds were being bypassed, the subjects had no way of telling. During the next eight hours, a battery of tests was used to assess the consequences of each mystery meal. Relying literally on their gut feelings, patients had to identify which of the liquid meals that had been poured down the naso-gastric tubes contained the food they couldn't tolerate. The results confirmed those of the previous experiments; between them the patients correctly identified ten of the twelve occasions on which they received the suspect foods, and eleven of the twelve occasions on which breakfast was harmless.

These precautions may seem rather elaborate. Why, for example, didn't Dr Hunter allow his subjects to eat the suspect foods in the usual way instead of having them flushed in this rather unpleasant manner through the nose? It seems to imply that irritable bowel patients can't be trusted to know their own minds – and bodies – or to tell the truth. In fact it was simply to ensure that the patients' suspicions about which foods caused their symptoms didn't bias their own perceptions. The taste of the food would, of course, have alerted them to what they were eating. As our states of mind have considerable effect on the activity of our guts, people who become mistakenly convinced that such and such a food causes them trouble are quite likely to make a self-fulfilling prophecy. If I believe fervently enough that eggs with brown shells make me ill, but eggs with white ones don't, the chances are that brown-shelled ones will indeed prove troublesome when I know I'm eating one. Only when I don't know the colour of the egg I've swallowed can I be certain that my suspicions are well-founded, and that my mind isn't simply lording it over my body. (For more on the theoretical basis of the way in which scientists and doctors conduct medical experiments, see the chapter on hypnosis, page 118.)

In Dr Hunter's experiments there was little doubt that many patients were responding badly to specific foods. His attempts to find out why were less conclusive. He was unable to unearth evidence that any of the various foods were activating the immune system. In other words, there was no reason to believe that this was an allergy in the strict sense of that word. He does have some general thoughts on the matter, and I'll be turning to those later.

Problems with food intolerance

As Dr Hunter himself admits, the use of exclusion diets in trying to pin down and overcome the cause of the irritable bowel syndrome is no easy option. However, experience has now taught him and his colleagues which foods are most likely to prove troublesome; so many patients are able to take some short cuts when finding out which things to avoid. Ninety per cent of patients who've used the exclusion diet are said still to be free of symptoms two years later – an impressive success rate.

Now for the bad news. I described this work as controversial because not everyone has managed to get such good results as Dr Hunter. There is, at present, no explanation for the discrepancies. One of the researchers who tried and failed to get the same success points out that a disproportionate number of Dr Hunter's patients appear to have had diarrhoea rather than constipation as their main symptom. Like many doctors he wonders if the IBS is really a collection of different disorders – in which case it might be that dietary causes are important in some patients, but not in all. Another attempt to test the food exclusion principle was carried out on patients who were also asked to undergo a psychiatric examination. A majority of them turned out to show evidence of minor psychiatric disorder. I'll be exploring this and similar findings in the next chapter.

Meanwhile the world turns; at the time of writing, the latest report to appear *does* provide support for the food intolerance theory. Dr Derek Jewell of the Radcliffe Infirmary in Oxford has studied a group of two hundred IBS patients who had failed to respond to drug treatment, a high fibre diet, and bulking agents: difficult cases, in other words. Each patient was asked to follow a diet limited to fresh meat, fish, vegetables, rice and products derived from goat, sheep or soya milk. If, at the end of three weeks, they had experienced no improvement, they were told that food intolerance was not the cause of the problem and that they could return to a normal diet. If they improved they then began, as in Dr Hunter's work, to reintroduce the foods one at a time in a set order. Each new food was tested for two days before the patient went on to the next. If a particular food was found to provoke IBS symptoms, it was left out of the diet.

Almost half the patients claimed that the exclusion diet did improve their condition. Three quarters of these were able to identify the foodstuffs which were troubling them. Most were intolerant of more than one food, and more than half listed between two and five. The 'top ten' were cheese, onions, milk, wheat, chocolate, butter, yoghourt, coffee, eggs and nuts. Patients who persevered with their diet were still keeping their disease in check when Dr Jewell completed the study – a period ranging from a few months to up to a year or two. The patients who'd shown no evidence of food intolerance meanwhile continued to fare as badly as ever.

Monitoring the muscles

Whenever a muscle contracts, it does so in response to electrical messages which travel along each of its component muscle fibres. As IBS patients have gut muscles which are very obviously contracting inappropriately, some researchers have looked for an inherent abnormality in the pattern of electrical activity within the muscles themselves. Like everything about the IBS, this turns out to be more complicated than you had hoped.

The smooth muscle of the gut displays two types of electrical activity. The first of these, known as the basic electrical rhythm (and also by several other names) shows itself as a series of waves of activity with a regularity which depends on where in the gut they are measured. In the colon there are two such electrical waves: one waxes and wanes about three times every minute. To put it more technically, it fluctuates at a rate of three cycles per second. The other and predominant rhythm is more than twice as frequent, having a periodicity of about six to nine cycles per second. The two may be superimposed on each other, and at times both disappear. In addition to these basic electrical rhythms there is another type of activity referred to as a spike. This brief and rapid rise and fall in the voltage within the muscle is comparable to the electrical message passing down a nerve, and is often but not always associated with a contraction of the muscle in which it's being recorded. Before saying – or more realistically guessing – how all this relates to the IBS, it's worth pausing briefly to describe how these measurements of electrical activity are made.

The electrical activity in a part of the body is recorded by attaching to it a suitable piece of metal called an electrode. This is then wired up to an instrument which can display the electrical pulses recorded in the form of a line (often using a pen moving over a paper strip) which 'wobbles' back and forth each time a wave or a spike reaches the electrode. In an electrocardiogram, for example, the object is to record the electrical activity of the muscles of the heart; so the electrodes are placed on the chest at the nearest point to the heart. Of course, much better recordings can be made if the electrodes are placed as close as possible to the muscles under study. Measuring the electrical activity in, say, the biceps of the arm is quite easy. These lie just beneath the skin. But the muscles of the gut are altogether less accessible. The only way to approach them is through – yes, once again I'm afraid – the anus and rectum.

The investigator inserts a sigmoidoscope to whatever distance from the end of the gut at which he wishes to make the measurements. Through this he then slides a wire with the electrode mounted on its tip. To obtain a good recording, the electrode has to be securely fixed to the tissue from which readings are to be taken. One way of doing this is to use an electrode in the form of a clip which can be attached to the lining of the gut. Another type relies on having a needle-like electrode projecting from the centre of a small rubber cup. When the cup has been manoeuvred into the correct position, suction is used to press it against the bowel wall – so forcing the electrode a couple of millimetres into the tissue. Sounds nasty – but it's quite painless. Once the electrodes are in place, the sigmoidoscope is withdrawn and recording can begin. I should say that this is a research technique; it's most unlikely to be used for routine diagnosis.

Researchers were naturally interested to find out if recordings made from the guts of IBS sufferers would differ at all from those made using healthy individuals. And they weren't disappointed. First to perform this experiment were some doctors at the University of Pennsylvania. The biggest difference they found was in the proportion of time for which the colon displayed the two basic electrical rhythms. The three-cycles-per-minute component accounted for four times as much of the basic electrical rhythm in IBS patients as in the healthy subjects. Here then, is a clear difference. But why should this difference lead to the symptoms of the irritable bowel syndrome?

One suggestion is that gut muscles which spend more of their time in the slow electrical wave state are more susceptible to other things – from emotions to hormones – which wouldn't otherwise prove troublesome. There's some indirect evidence for this. Another group of American researchers, this time working on healthy volunteers, tried out the effect of injections of a drug called pentagastrin. This is a synthetic equivalent of a hormone called gastrin which stimulates the secretion of gastric juices by the stomach. The Americans found that the effects of pentagastrin depended on which type of electrical activity the colon happened to be displaying when the subject was given the injection. If the predominant basic electrical rhythm was the slow type, the hormone had little effect. However, if the pentagastrin injection happened to be given at a time when the slower (three-cycles-per-minute) waves predominated, these became more pronounced. And this change was then followed by a marked increase in the contractions of the gut's muscle: just the sort of activity which might lead to the symptoms of an irritable bowel.

Here, then, is the germ of another explanation: that people with the IBS have gut muscles with an undue amount of a particular type of electrical rhythm. This rhythm, so the argument goes, is associated with a tendency to respond to things which wouldn't otherwise induce much activity in the gut. You can find an analogy in people who suffer from hay fever. Although their sensitivity to pollen is there all the time, for most of the year they don't look or behave any differently from anyone else. Only in summer, and even then only intermittently, do they encounter the pollen which makes them sneeze. No pollen, no trouble. And so it may be for IBS patients who succeed in identifying their equivalent to the hay fever sufferer's pollen grains. Specific foods could be one such factor: stress another.

If the root of the IBS patients' problems do indeed lie in the electrical activity of their gut muscles, what happens when their symptoms respond to a treatment such as bran? The answer appears to be ... nothing. Some doctors in Liverpool have measured the electrical activity of the gut in IBS patients before and after treatment. Even in patients whose symptoms cleared up, the electrical activity remained the same. This, of course, is more or less what you'd expect if a treatment is doing no more than counteracting whatever is provoking the symptoms. The underlying sensitivity would remain. And this would explain why patients so often relapse. If an electrical disturbance is indeed at the root of the syndrome, only a treatment which corrects that disturbance could really be called a cure. For the moment, there's much about this topic which remains controversial – not least because some researchers have failed to find anything electrically different about IBS patients. But that seems to be par for the course in research on this difficult disease. Someone reports a new research finding; someone else repeats the work and gets a different result. Then a third researcher enters the fray and seems to confirm the original finding. And so it goes on.

A disorder of smooth muscle?

Most of the research on IBS patients has focussed on the large bowel. However, patients can also be shown to have disturbances in the workings of the small bowel and even the oesophagus. This has prompted some doctors to wonder if the IBS is one manifestation of a more generalized disturbance. Smooth muscle, the type found in the gut, also appears in other locations around the body. The IBS might be just one instance – albeit the most clear cut – of what is really a bodywide disturbance of smooth muscle.

To investigate this possibility, Dr Peter Whorwell of the University of Manchester asked some of the IBS patients attending his clinic to take part in an investigation of their bladder muscles. He found that half of the IBS patients had evidence of bladder problems, and a greatly disproportionate number had a condition called 'detrusor instability'. The detrusor muscle is a component of the wall of the bladder which plays an important part both in keeping it closed, and in emptying it at appropriate times. Detrusor instability is a disturbance of the smooth muscle of the bladder which is known to give rise to frequency and urgency. The finding that IBS patients are so much more likely to suffer from it is certainly consistent with the notion that the IBS is one of perhaps many adverse consequences of a widespread smooth muscle abnormality. But the evidence remains circumstantial.

Hormones

At least ten hormones are known to have an effect on the activity of the gut, some inhibiting it, others stimulating it to more active movement. So could it be that the irritable bowel syndrome is a result of some kind of hormonal disturbance? It's tempting to think so because the main stimulus to the release of gut hormones into the bloodstream is eating – and it's eating which provokes the most severe abdominal pain in many IBS patients.

One of the most tantalizing studies was performed about fifteen years ago by doctors in Bristol. They injected twenty patients with a hormone called cholecystokinin. The main action of this hormone is to prompt the gallbladder to pour bile into the intestine. The researchers found that eight of their patients experienced a marked increase in gut activity. These eight patients were the very ones whose pain was usually brought on by eating. Moreover four of these eight reported that the hormone provoked a pain indistinguishable from their IBS pain. Cholecystokinin output is especially associated with meals containing large amounts of fat and protein – and half of the eight patients said that their IBS symptoms were most often brought on by fried foods and fatty meat, especially pork.

Alas, the picture becomes a little less clear cut when you discover that some patients demonstrated little or no response to the hormone, while others receiving the same dose showed a massive increase in gut activity. Moreoever, the measurement of this and other hormone levels in people with and without the IBS has not revealed any consistent differences. So if hormones have anything at all to do with the irritable bowel syndrome, it seems more likely that what is abnormal is not the output of those hormones but some kind of over-reaction to them. Even so, this is pure guesswork, and too little is known about the hormones of the gut to make any judgement. Ignorance in this area is profound even by the standards prevailing more generally in matters concerning the IBS.

Life in the gut

A lot of researchers have commented on the number of IBS patients whose symptoms seem to date from the time of an intestinal infection, or an operation, or from various other forms of medical treatment. What all these events have in common is that they are capable of bringing about a change in the type of bacteria living in the gut. This opens up yet another theory about the irritable bowel syndrome: that it's not only how you live which counts, but also what is living within you.

This is another idea which has been pursued by Dr Hunter at Addenbrooke's Hospital. He discovered that many of the patients themselves believed that their problems were attributable to a specific event: a course of antibiotics, a gastrointestinal infection, or an operation. Half the patients who mentioned an operation were women who thought it was something to do with the hysterectomies they'd had. Dr Hunter decided to follow the progress of a group of women undergoing this operation. With the co-operation of his gynaecological colleagues, he asked women being admitted to the hospital for a hysterectomy to fill in a questionnaire intended to find out if they already suffered from the symptoms of the irritable bowel. Any who did were eliminated from the study. This left 113 patients.

During the surgery, roughly three-fifths of these women

were given an antibiotic called metronidazole. This is intended to prevent infections which might otherwise result from the operation. Some surgeons use antibiotics as a matter of course; others don't believe they're necessary. For Dr Hunter's purposes, these two forms of routine practice constituted an experiment: one in which he was able to compare the outcome as far as the irritable bowel syndrome was concerned. A further questionnaire sent out a couple of months later revealed that thirteen of the womem had developed IBS symptoms since their operations. All but one of these thirteen were among the 60 per cent of the original group who had received the antibiotic.

Eager to test the antibiotic connection more thoroughly, Dr Hunter and his colleagues next organized a second and larger experiment. This one involved women who were due to have a hysterectomy performed by one of the gynaecologists who did not normally prescribe an antibiotic, but who didn't have any objection to some of his patients receiving one anyway. And that is how things were arranged. Half the women, chosen at random, were given one dose of metronidazole antibiotic before the operation at the time of their premed, one on the evening of the operation day, and three further doses at twelve-hourly intervals. Some of the women who hadn't been allocated to the antibiotic group were later judged to need one. So the antibiotic group grew larger than its non-antibiotic counterpart. In the end sixty-two patients received antibiotics; of these seven developed IBS symptoms. Twenty patients did not receive antibiotics; none developed IBS symptoms.

Why the difference? Why should a course of antibiotics provoke this disorder? Dr Hunter believes that it's not the antibiotics themselves which are important, but the effect they have on our internal menagerie: on the body's bacteria. All of us have vast numbers of microbes living quite happily inside our guts, doing no harm and in some cases doing some good – remember the bacteria of the large intestine which break down otherwise indigestible materials. A dose of antibiotic flooding through the bowel may be unavoidable if the body has been invaded by disease-producing bacteria (the 'bad guys'); but, although some antibiotics have a degree of selectivity, they can't be guaranteed to knock out only these unwelcome microbes. In fact many antibiotics are chosen precisely because they have a broad spectrum of activity. This can be helpful when, for example, the doctor doesn't know exactly what species or strain of bacterium has to be eliminated. The drawback of this shotgun tactic is that many of the 'good guys' are hit just as hard.

If a dose of antibiotic does eliminate most of the bacteria living in the gut, one of two things may happen. With luck, any new bacteria which colonize the gut (there's no shortage; we swallow vast numbers of microbes all the time) will live as harmoniously with their host as did the previous inhabitants. But this may not be what happens; the virgin territories of the bacterially denuded bowel may instead be invaded by a slightly different range of bacterial species. The owner of the intestine may be less well adjusted to the new inhabitants of his internal zoo. The details of what could happen under these circumstances are still a matter of guesswork; but suppose the new occupants of the bowel have a different way of breaking down the foodstuffs in which they find themselves floating. As a consequence they might produce some different chemicals. And if some of these alien chemicals happen to be materials to which that particular person's gut reacts badly, their effect may be such as to provoke the symptoms which we recognize as an irritable bowel. Similar changes in the types of bacteria living in the gut – the gut 'flora' to use the technical and, for once, rather appealing term – could also be induced by other medical procedures including radiotherapy or perhaps even an anaesthetic.

Diet and the gut microbes

It's now possible to see how diet might fit into the picture. As long as someone eats only foodstuffs which encourage the growth of those types of bacteria which don't produce any chemicals to which his particular gut reacts adversely, there is no problem. But if that person changes his diet, a different set of nutrients will be available to the gut bacteria. Two things could happen: they might start to produce a chemical which they weren't previously making; or, a strain of some relatively disagreeable bacterium which was previously being held in check might begin to proliferate and overwhelm its more benign counterparts. Dr Hunter has some direct experimental evidence for the second of these two processes.

Working with microbiologist colleagues, he arranged for a microbial analysis of the faecal flora of a group of IBS patients known to be intolerant of, among other things, wheat. The aim of such an analysis is to find out what types of bacteria are living in the bowel; it's done by culturing a stool sample and examining the bacterial colonies which begin to grow. Dr Hunter arranged for one analysis to be carried out forty-eight hours before, and another seventy-two hours after the patients had eaten some wheat in the form of bread. Following this food, several of them showed a marked change in the types of bacteria predominating in their gut flora; indeed, in a couple of patients the number of one particular variety of bacterium shot up more than a hundredfold. This was a very small study; but it does seem to suggest that changes in the food eaten can bring about marked alterations to the population of bacteria living within the bowel.

The next step must be to define these changes more thoroughly, and then to find out which of the chemicals being produced by the gut bacteria might be causing the IBS symptoms. Unfortunately this is extremely difficult, not least because of the bewildering complexity of the soup of chemicals which comprise the gut contents. If Dr Hunter's theory is correct, it might open the way to some new treatments for the irritable bowel. If the obnoxious chemical could be identified, scientists might be able to develop a drug which would selectively inhibit whatever harmful action it was having on the body. More ambitiously still, it might be possible to manipulate the gut flora by creating an environment in which the most desirable bacteria would be best able to flourish. If a change of diet couldn't be used to achieve this end, swallowing a drug of some kind might again be the way to create the desired environment.

It's easy enough to see how the food intolerance theory could account for some of the other characteristics of IBS patients. It could, for example, explain why some respond adversely to fibre while for others, fibre effectively relieves their symptoms. Food intolerance is also compatible with the observation that IBS patients have trouble with smooth muscles in parts of the body outside the gut. Toxic or poisonous chemicals may exert their most immediate and dramatic effects on the gut itself; but once they've been absorbed and passed into the bloodstream, they can affect organs elsewhere in the body. The fault, however, would lie not in the smooth muscle itself, but in the chemicals which were adversely affecting it.

Hyperventilation

Dr Hunter does not suggest that all the patients coming to him with the irritable bowel syndrome are suffering from food intolerance. In the Cambridge area where he works, he reckons that this accounts for about half the IBS patients attending his clinic. He thinks that as many as another quarter of his patients are suffering from hyperventilation. This is one of the few explanations for the IBS which seem not to have been widely discussed in the medical literature.

Hyperventilation means exactly what you might deduce from the word itself: that is, breathing too much. On first hearing, the notion of 'breathing too much' seems distinctly odd. Breathing, after all, serves two purposes. First and most obviously there's the need to supply the surfaces of the lungs with fresh oxygen which can diffuse into their fine blood vessels, and so be carried throughout the body. Second, the carbon dioxide produced by all living tissues and absorbed by the blood has to diffuse in the opposite direction: that is, from the blood vessels, into the lungs, and so out of the body. If you exercise you breathe harder: more oxygen is required and more carbon dioxide is produced. That said, it's still not immediately obvious why breathing more than you need to at any particular moment should be bad for you. If extra oxygen is brought to the bloodstream and more carbon dioxide is removed from it, can these events be anything but good? The answer is that they can – at least in the case of the carbon dioxide.

Although carbon dioxide is a waste product, the body is adapted to expect a certain amount of it to be present in the blood at any particular time. If you breathe more than you need to, the carbon dioxide level rapidly falls to a lower level than normal, and this alters the acidity of the blood. This in turn makes nerve cells more excitable, and narrows the vessels which carry blood to the brain, so reducing its oxygen supply. The outcome is a startlingly wide range of symptoms including pains in the chest, abnormal heart rhythms, visual and hearing disturbances, vertigo, muscular cramps and sudden losses of strength, fatigue, difficulty in swallowing and breathing, sweating, fainting, headaches, anxiety, dizziness, panic attacks ... the list could go on. The significance of all this as far as the IBS is concerned is that the list includes pain in the stomach, diarrhoea, bloating, and belching.

Hyperventilation is best known – in so far as most people have ever heard of it – as an alternative explanation for the multiplicity of problems encountered by the few but much publicized individuals who believe themselves to be allergic to most of the synthetic chemicals of the twentieth century: the 'total allergy syndrome', as it's been dubbed. Some doctors sceptical of this explanation have suggested that what really happens is that certain individuals form an erroneous but deeply held belief that they are unduly sensitive to their environment; this, understandably, makes them nervous and anxious – one consequence of which is that they breathe more deeply or more rapidly. This induces some of the symptoms which they fear. These symptoms are then attributed to the presumed allergy – and so the original fears are apparently confirmed. This, of course, serves to reinforce them. One simple way of checking if people's symptoms are a consequence of hyperventilation is to have them breathe in and out of a large paper bag: in other words, to rebreathe the same air several times over. The rising concentration of carbon dioxide in the bag will rapidly bring about a corresponding increase in the amount of carbon dioxide in the blood. The symptoms should become less severe. Clearly this can't be kept up for long enough to find out if IBS symptoms would disappear; the only thing one would achieve is asphyxiation! But anyone whose IBS is accompanied by some of the more acute symptoms listed above might give this a whirl and see what happens.

If hyperventilation really is the cause of at least some cases of the irritable bowel syndrome, what can be done? Simply telling people to breathe less deeply or less often may not be a great deal of help, because most hyperventilators aren't aware that there is anything unusual about their pattern of breathing. A physiotherapist may be able to help; and hypnosis is another way of tackling the problem. One or two doctors have used a dual approach, combining what is known as 'autohypnosis' with instructions on how to breathe correctly. While the patients are hypnotized, the therapist teaches them a specific signal which they will later be able to use to put themselves into a hypnotic state at any time they choose. This signal will only work if the person himself uses it, and the 'autohypnotic' state so induced will last only about twenty minutes. At the end of this time subjects will come out of it of their own accord. When any symptoms which might be due to hyperventilation are felt to be coming on, a quick 'burst' of this treatment may help. (There's more on hypnosis in Chapter 8.)

In concert with this approach it makes sense to teach a more relaxed form of breathing which uses the diaphragm rather than the chest. To learn this, the patient places one hand just above the belly button, and the other flat on the chest. On each inward breath, the hand resting on the chest should feel no particular movement, while the hand resting against the upper abdomen should be pushed forward. This happens because the diaphragm is a layer of muscular tissue which lies above the abdominal cavity (which contains the intestines and most of the rest of the internal organs), but below the thoracic cavity which houses the lungs. At rest the diaphragm projects upwards like a shallow dome. When its muscles contract,the dome flattens, and drags air down into the lungs. This flattening also puts a downward pressure on the stomach – which consequently bulges forward. Most hyperventilators do most of their breathing by using their chest muscles; they have to learn to make more use of the diaphragm. Most people in a hypnotic state will automatically breathe using the diaphragm.

There is, of course, a whole raft of other factors contributing to the irritable bowel syndrome which have so far been mentioned only in passing; these are mood, emotion, psychiatric disorders, stresses – and the IBS sufferer's response to them. The contentious topic of psychological factors – the root of much of the difficulty which patients face when they seek treatment – will be tackled in the next chapter.

4   In the Mind . . .
       and the Body

On earth there is nothing great but man;
in man there is nothing great but mind.

'Lectures on Metaphysics',
Sir William Hamilton

'It's all in your mind' is one of the most irritating, most
insulting things you can say to people experiencing what
are, to them, unequivocally physical symptoms. Their
annoyance is wholly justified when, as is often the case,
the comment is patronizing, or meant as a put-down: as
a way of saying, 'There's nothing *really* wrong with you.
Pull yourself together and stop complaining.' Regrettably
this *is* more or less what some doctors mean when they
use the phrase, or others like it. And yet there are circumstances in which doctor and patient can agree that a
particular problem really is wholly in the mind. The most
dramatic and clear-cut instance is surely the phantom
limb phenomenon experienced by some people who've
had an arm or a leg amputated. If they close their eyes,
the amputated limb feels as if it's still there. It may itch;
worse, and more commonly, it feels painful. Yet when the
amputee opens his eyes, he knows every bit as surely as

his doctor that the limb has gone. The paradox is easily explained. The pain is real. Its source, though, lies not in a frostbitten toe or a broken shinbone but in the amputee's own head: inside the part of the brain responsible for creating the perception or state of mind which we call 'pain'.

In the case of a phantom limb, the brain misperceives physical reality. But that's merely the passive end of this troublesome spectrum. The brain can also – equally tiresomely and inappropriately – alter reality by inducing physical disease in the body. The most familiar example of this is the link between stress and heart disease. Its true importance – in other words how many people who die of heart disease would not have done so if they'd been living an unstressed life – is impossible to estimate. Psychosomatic factors, as they're known, seldom operate in isolation from diet, smoking and the other risk factors known to be associated with heart disease. In some individuals, stress may be no more than the trigger which precipitates the final crisis. More controversially, there has been much discussion of a possible link between stressful life events and certain forms of cancer. Some of those who've become convinced of the existence of such a link have even tried to turn it to therapeutic advantage. They treat cancer by techniques which rely on the use of the mind to mobilize the body's natural capacity to attack its own tumour cells. In one such technique, called visualization, cancer patients are instructed to create a vivid mental image of their tumour as under attack by the cells of their immune defence system. The hope is that by having patients concentrate their conscious thoughts on one of the body's healing processes, they can actually spur that process to greater achievements.

While there isn't yet a great deal of hard evidence that this particular technique works, there is now a mass of evidence – some anecdotal, some from careful experiments – that the mind can influence the body in all sorts of ways. To put it in the homeliest terms possible, you really do become more susceptible to infectious diseases when you're feeling 'run down'. And given the extent to which states of mind influence all sorts of chemical and other processes going on in the body, it's hard to imagine why we should ever have doubted this. The difficulty which does remain is knowing how to exploit this realization for purposes of treatment: to 'think your way to better health', as it were.

Gut reactions

There is, fortunately, one matter about which everyone can agree: that certain states of mind can have a profound effect on what happens in the gut. Young policemen and women called for the first time to sort out the carnage of a major road accident may vomit; soldiers waiting to go into battle have been known to lose control of their anal sphincters; pulp fiction abounds with characters whose 'stomachs turn over' or whose 'bowels seem to turn to liquid' when they're shocked or startled; and all of us have experienced the butterflies in the stomach, the lump in the throat, or the sudden desire to visit the lavatory which often precedes a speech, an interview, or some other such dreaded engagement.

The evolutionary logic of these gut reactions is by no means clear – which is odd because many of the changes associated with fear clearly do serve a useful purpose. The 'fight or flight response' is a shorthand way of describing the set of bodily changes provoked by circumstances in which we know that survival depends on holding our ground and doing battle, or running like the devil to escape. Once our brains have become alerted to the danger, they use the autonomic nervous system to instruct many of the body's organ systems to undertake a series of actions which are then reinforced by an outpouring of certain hormones, notably adrenaline. Among the consequences of this flurry of nervous and chemical messages is the diversion of blood from the stomach and the bowels to the muscles. Under normal circumstances the gut needs a rich blood supply to take up the nutrients absorbed through the lining of the intestine. But if the issue is one of immediate survival, it's clearly sensible to put digestion on the backburner, and make full use of the blood system for transporting oxygen to the muscles. There's little sense in being well-nourished but dead. (Incidentally, while the condemned man may have eaten a hearty breakfast, it's unlikely that much of it was absorbed before the moment of execution.) About all one can say of butterflies in the stomach and the rest of these irksome symptoms is that they must be the side effects of some process which is serving a greater purpose.

Understanding the gut-brain connection

In trying to understand the link between mind and body which is undoubtedly playing a part in the irritable bowel syndrome, a series of questions have to be answered. Easily the most obvious is the extent to which IBS patients are psychologically, emotionally or by virtue of something about their personalities, a group apart. Many researchers believe that your risk of heart disease is affected by certain characteristics of outlook and behaviour which they label 'Type A' and 'Type B'. Is there, similarly, an IBS-prone personality? Some forms of mental disturbance seem to produce a characteristic set of physical symptoms; so could the IBS be a manifestation of some form of neurotic illness, for example, depression or anxiety? And then there's the issue of cause and effect: if IBS patients are psychologically or emotionally different from the rest of the population, are their IBS symptoms one manifestation of this difference? Or is any psychological difference a consequence of the distress induced by the physical symptoms, and not the cause of it? Doctors have been asking these questions for several decades – and all too often coming up with contradictory answers.

Most researchers seem to have assumed that psychological factors play a part of some kind in the illness. The early and still much-quoted work of Drs Chaudhary and Truelove (see page 22) describes three quarters of their patients as being subject to at least one such psychological factor. Other doctors have taken the wholly unequivocal view that the irritable bowel syndrome is the bodily manifestation of what is, at root, an emotional disorder. Back in the early seventies, for example, an Australian gastroenterologist, Dr Ian Hislop, studied almost seventy patients who had been referred for a specialist opinion on their gut problems, and had been diagnosed as suffering from the IBS. He compared them with another group of people (some healthy, and some attending the hospital casualty department for minor injuries), none of whom had gut problems. He found that the IBS patients were anything from three to seven times as likely to suffer from one or more of the following: fatigue, depression, insomnia, bouts of weeping, anorexia and suicidal behaviour. A disproportionate number of the patients were having to cope with marriage problems, and more of them had had emotionally disturbed childhoods.

Having carefully totted up all these differences, Dr Hislop goes on to note that many authorities on psychiatric illness have pointed out how clinically depressed patients may perceive bodily symptoms as their chief complaint. These symptoms not infrequently include abdominal pain, nausea, vomiting and constipation. It's this which leads Dr Hislop to conclude, with apparent confidence, that the irritable bowel syndrome is actually a psychiatric disorder. Indeed, a succession of studies carried out over some fifty years have found that IBS patients are more than averagely anxious or depressed. But how much do these findings tell us about the mass of IBS patients? Not a great deal, perhaps. After all, the majority of people with IBS symptoms do not consult a doctor. Therefore the individuals who've taken part in some of these research studies might not be a representative cross-section of all sufferers. It's easy to see that IBS sufferers with physical symptoms alone would be less likely to take their problems to a doctor than would others with those same symptoms plus an emotional disturbance of some kind. Likewise people who are, of their nature, highly strung might be more likely to visit the doctor than others with equally troubling physical symptoms but who happen to be of a less nervous disposition.

Illness behaviour

Some researchers have made a determined effort to overcome these uncertainties. One of the more interesting attempts was made by American psychologist Dr William Whitehead and his colleagues. They started from the premise that there is what they call a 'social dimension' to any experience of illness which determines how an individual perceives and interprets bodily changes, and what he does about them. They quote some examples. We all know people who are chronically ill, but who deny that there is anything wrong with them. They may decline all offers of help, refuse to see a doctor, and fail to accept any treatment which is offered. At the other extreme are people preoccupied with their ailments, who repeatedly visit the doctor, and who seem to experience bodily discomfort which is out of all proportion to what might be expected of whatever disease they have. The jargon term for this is 'chronic illness behaviour'. But why should some people feel the need to behave in this way? When two men using hammers accidentally hit their thumbs with more or less the same degree of force, one may curse his bad luck, perhaps suck the injured digit, but then get on with the job; the other may stop work altogether until the fuss and sympathy of his spouse finally persuades him to resume. Why? Psychologists argue that one of the factors which determine how we respond to an accident or an illness is what we've learned by seeing how others react.

As Dr Whitehead points out, biofeedback techniques (see page 135) have revealed how it's possible to influence physiological processes – including the secretion of acid by the stomach, and the activity of the gut – which aren't normally under conscious control. Having offered this reminder that even apparently uncontrollable bodily functions can to some degree be influenced, Dr Whitehead goes on to argue that, 'by analogy, a parent might inadvertently train abnormal physiological responses by attending to a child and allowing him to stay home from school when he complains of a stomach ache'. This is the theory of 'learned illness behaviour'; it maintains that certain functional disorders serve the purpose of attracting extra attention and sympathy, and of allowing patients who experience them to avoid disagreeable social or work obligations. In the particular example quoted, the child soon realizes that developing a stomach ache earns the highly valued reward of not having to go to school; and once this pattern of using an illness to achieve a desired end has become established, it continues through into adult life.

This is not, let's be clear, anything to do with malingering; there is no conscious attempt to fake symptoms. The symptoms are real – but induced by a mind which has learned how to create a situation which the patient may not consciously desire but which, subconsciously, may nevertheless suit him or her quite well.

Even as I write this, I can feel the hackles of IBS sufferers rising. How dare anyone suggest that they are behaving in such a manipulative fashion, even if it is without their having consciously willed it. I have a certain sympathy with people who feel outraged by suggestions like this. To be honest, I too would be sorely tempted to walk out on any doctor who tried to describe an illness of mine in these terms. There are moments at which a wholly objective, totally dispassionate demeanour is difficult to maintain! In fairness, though, there is some evidence to support the theory of learned illness behaviour in the irritable bowel syndrome. So before you dismiss this view as unjustifiably impertinent, judge the evidence for yourself.

Dr Whitehead's study was cleverly constructed. He first looked for people with two diseases: the IBS, and also peptic ulcer disease. He chose this second one because, although related to the IBS by virtue of being another gastrointestinal disorder, it does involve a definite organic change. I say he 'looked' for subjects because he didn't choose his subjects solely from among those who had taken their complaint to a doctor. Instead he used people drawn at random from the Cincinnati telephone directory. They were first contacted by letter (a sensible precaution: strangers who ring up unexpectedly to enquire about people's bowel habits are likely to invite the attention of the police) and then telephoned by trained interviewers who asked them some eighty questions about their health, the use they made of medical facilities, and their early experiences in relation to childhood colds and 'flu. Of the eight hundred or so people contacted, 8 per cent turned out to have the symptoms of the IBS; a further 10 per cent had been diagnosed by their doctor as having an ulcer; and the rest were normal as far as these two complaints were concerned.

When the researchers analysed the answers they'd been given, they found that people with the IBS were more likely than people without this disorder to have had two or more colds during the previous year; to believe that their colds were more serious than those of other people; to go to a doctor when suffering from a cold or 'flu instead of treating it themselves; and to have missed work or changed their activities because of physical illness on more than four days during the previous year. As far as the questions about childhood illness were concerned, people falling into the categories just listed were also more likely to have had parents who showed them extra consideration when ill by giving them special foods, toys or other gifts.

You can probably guess (perhaps while gnashing your teeth if you're an IBS sufferer) what conclusions Dr Whitehead drew from his study: that a history, dating from childhood, of receiving social rewards for illness predisposes one to the development of the irritable bowel syndrome in later life. People on the other hand with ulcer disease – an organic, not a functional disorder – are no different in respect of their childhood experiences and their adult behaviour from the rest of the population. The really irritating feature of theories like this is that they're difficult to refute. And no one likes the notion that their autonomy has been compromised, especially in such a self-serving manner as this.

Of course, it could be argued that people with the irritable bowel syndrome are simply predisposed to suffer more illness, more seriously, and more often than the rest of the population, and that it's nothing to do with childhood learning. Dr Whitehead rejects this explanation on the grounds that most IBS patients are otherwise physically healthy. Even so, the possibility of a genuine difference can't be entirely ruled out.

A few researchers have tried to find out if there's anything distinctive about the personalities of IBS sufferers. Some researchers in London asked a group of IBS patients to complete standard personality inventory tests, including the one devised by the psychologist Professor Hans Eysenck. The subjects turned out to have personalities more characterized by neuroticism than were those of healthy subjects. In general their scores tended to lie somewhere between those of healthy people, and those of patients diagnosed as suffering from explicitly neurotic disorders. As ever, though, it's difficult to draw any very definite conclusions from the work.

Who goes to the doctor?

Several research groups have tried to find out if all IBS sufferers are equally likely to take their symptoms to the doctor, or if some have a psychological predisposition which makes it more probable that they will do so. One such study comes from New Zealand where three researchers compared the psychological state of IBS sufferers being seen in a hospital outpatient department with, firstly, IBS sufferers who hadn't reported their illness and, secondly, otherwise healthy people. They use standard questionnaires to assess their subjects' states of mind.

They found that IBS sufferers – both those who had sought treatment and those who hadn't – showed more 'somatic distress' than non-IBS subjects. Somatic distress is a term used to describe the concern and worry associated with a variety of minor physical complaints such as headaches, breathlessness and palpitations. That IBS sufferers should experience more of this kind of thing is hardly surprising. Anyone who suffers from a chronic and painful condition like the IBS might well be expected to find additional, non-gut symptoms harder to bear than people not so afflicted. You could say that they've become sensitized to the presence of other minor maladies. However, there was no discernible difference between IBS patients and non-patient IBS sufferers. None of the three groups of subjects showed any major differences in anxiety or depression. In short, the New Zealand doctors weren't able to say why the people they'd worked with either did or did not seek a doctor's help for their irritable bowels.

A more recent study – this too from the aforementioned Dr William Whitehead – reaches very different conclusions. Readers who are still smarting over Dr Whitehead's theory of learned illness behaviour may be inclined to forgive him a little when they've chewed over the findings of this later study. It makes no reference to learned illness behaviour, or indeed to any of the earlier work.

On this occasion he had set out to test a number of ideas about the irritable bowel syndrome – but the one relevant to this particular part of the debate is what's known as the 'self-selection' hypothesis. This is simply a shorthand way of describing one of the possible explanations for the disproportionate number of IBS patients who seem to be psychologically disturbed. It suggests that while psychological distress doesn't *cause* the syndrome, IBS sufferers who also happen to be psychologically distressed are more likely to seek help for their physical symptoms. There's a parallel here with blood pressure. It's known that people who are being treated for high blood pressure have more symptoms of psychological distress than people who are newly detected by random screening. The inference is not that psychological factors cause high blood pressure, but that psychologically disturbed people are more likely to visit the doctor for all sorts of reasons, thereby increasing the likelihood that their high blood pressure will have been noticed and dealt with.

Dr Whitehead – who does show considerable experimental ingenuity – tested the self-selection hypothesis by comparing several groups of subjects. These included IBS patients attending a clinic for their disorder; and also IBS sufferers who had never sought medical help. (On this occasion Dr Whitehead didn't use the Cincinnati telephone directory. Instead he asked the directors of churchwomen's societies and charities to provide subjects in exchange for a donation payable on completion of each questionnaire!)

He was also interested in people with another bowel disturbance, lactose intolerance (see page 36). The standard way of identifying such people is known as a hydrogen breath test. Subjects are asked to fast overnight, and then given a specified quantity of lactose to drink. At hourly intervals over the next three hours the researchers collect samples of each subject's breath and test it for hydrogen. The principle behind this test is very simple. If the person who's swallowed the lactose lacks the enzyme required to digest it, the stuff will pass through the small intestine (in which it would otherwise be broken down and absorbed) and on into the large intestine. Here it will be broken down by bacteria – a process which leads to the release of, among other things, hydrogen. This passes into the bloodstream and reaches the lungs – where it diffuses out into the air which the subject then exhales. As with the IBS patients, Dr Whitehead had a group of people who'd attended a clinic on account of their lactose intolerance, and others who had never sought treatment but who had come to light through tests conducted on the invaluable church and charity volunteers.

All groups filled in detailed questionnaires designed to probe various elements of their states of mind. These measured all sorts of things including their level of anxiety, depression, paranoia, hostility and obsessive-compulsiveness. The results showed that previously unidentified

IBS sufferers showed no more psychological distress than did normal healthy individuals. But patients attending the clinic for their IBS showed more psychological symptoms than either group. In other words, the findings back the self-selection hypothesis: that while the irritable bowel syndrome itself isn't associated with psychological abnormalities, people who seek help for it *are* psychologically distinct. Something in their mood and outlook prompts them in particular to go to the doctor seeking help. (So doctors who draw the conclusion that *all* IBS sufferers share these characteristics are being misled.)

On then to the results of the tests carried out on people with lactose intolerance. The pattern was pretty much the same. Patients who had sought out treatment for their lactose intolerance had more symptoms of psychological distress than individuals with the disorder who were identified for the first time by Dr Whitehead's tests. This is important because although lactose intolerance is responsible for symptoms not unlike those of the IBS, there is no suggestion in this case of a psychological origin; indeed, the symptoms have a clear organic cause. This demonstrates that there is nothing contradictory about the suggestion that the irritable bowel syndrome might have a physical origin, yet only be brought to the attention of the doctor if the patient happens to be of a certain psychological make-up. This seems to be precisely what happens in the case of another organic disorder: that is, lactose intolerance.

Dr Whitehead is not, of course, suggesting that it's *only* patients of a certain psychological disposition who complain to the doctor about their symptoms. Severity too could well be another factor; indeed studies by other researchers have demonstrated that severity, especially pain, is something which prompts sufferers to seek medical advice.

Another report dating from about the same time as

the one just described puts a rather intriguing gloss on the outlook and behaviour of those people with the irritable bowel syndrome who choose not to seek medical help. A group of doctors and psychologists from North Carolina found that, compared with IBS patients, people in this category worried less about their health in general, showed more ability to cope with life, and had greater psychological stability when under stress. These IBS sufferers had clearly adapted to their illness.

The role of life events

Returning to the IBS sufferers who do decide to seek medical help: what prompts them to go to the doctor? Do they finally become weary of irksome bowel disturbances which have dragged on for years? Or is the decision to seek help prompted by some specific life crisis, or a change in the sufferer's emotional or psychological state? According to one authority, there was an increase in the prevalence of the irritable bowel syndrome during the last war. This could, presumably, be attributed to stress.

A few years ago, in an attempt to probe these links in more detail, a group of researchers in Edinburgh carried out detailed interviews with patients referred by GPs for specialist advice from a hospital gastrointestinal clinic. About three quarters of the patients were suffering from a functional disorder of the gut, principally the IBS. As they left the consulting room, they were approached and asked to co-operate in the study. Most agreed. Interviews were then used to build up a complete picture of the onset and duration of the problem, the nature and timing of any life events or major difficulties which had occurred during the previous six months, and any psychological or psychiatric disorders from which the patients were suffering.

Finding out, with the required reliability, if the subjects had endured any significant unpleasant life event involved more than merely asking them if they could indeed recall anything of that nature. Each one was presented with a list of commonly encountered life situations or events, and then closely questioned about any which they or people close to them had experienced. Each event could be categorized by the researchers as having one or more of six qualities or 'dimensions': threat; personal loss; hopelessness; uncertainty of outcome and so on. The death of a parent, for example, might involve two of these dimensions: loss and hopelessness.

As things turned out it's difficult to feel that all this detailed analysis was really worth the effort. Anxiety-provoking life events seemed to have featured in the lives of about a third of the patients studied – and the proportion was similar in patients attending the clinic for organic as opposed to functional disorders. Only when a life situation provoked a defined anxiety disorder did it seem to bear some direct relation to the onset of an irritable bowel. Other researchers who have tried this kind of exercise have come to a variety of conclusions: some have found that upsetting events *do* seem to precede (and, by implication, directly or indirectly create the circumstances which lead to) patients' decisions to attend a clinic. Others report no evidence of a causal link. Rather more encouragingly, Dr Chaudhary and his colleague looked at the effect of a major life change for the better (job, marriage, or whatever) among those of their patients in whom they believed that psychological factors were involved in provoking the IBS symptoms. They found that the outlook for patients who had experienced such a change became significantly better. So, *if* stress is playing a part, the harm it does can also be undone.

The Edinburgh study proved rather more positive when its organizers looked at the psychiatric state of the patients who took part. By the definitions they were using, a third of those who were interviewed could be said to have a psychiatric problem – and all but one of these individuals were in the 'functional' as opposed to the 'organic' bowel disorder category. A similar link was found when the researchers looked back at their subjects' past psychiatric history. More than half of the IBS-type patients had suffered from a psychiatric illness; that was four times the number of organic disorder patients who had done so. So non-organic disorders of the gut did here seem to be linked to the sufferers' states of mind.

Confused and confusing . . .

If the picture of the link between the mind and the gut which has so far emerged seems to be both confused and confusing, I can only say that that is more or less how many doctors also view it. A caustic review of the published work in this field, which appeared some five years ago, concluded that many of the research studies which had appeared (and still were appearing) had used unreliable methods of measuring their subjects' supposed psychiatric symptoms, or had used reliable measures inappropriately, or had failed to select subjects according to strict criteria – and had sometimes drawn the wrong conclusions from the data collected!

The authors of this review were two psychiatrists, Drs Creed and Guthrie, of the University Department of Psychiatry at Manchester Royal Infirmary. Having applauded their critical analysis of the attempts which have been made to identify the psychological factors in the IBS, it's worth reporting the findings of the studies which they themselves identify, Which? style, as 'best buys'. They picked out just two which met their strict criteria. Both suggest that 40-50 per cent of the patients referred to gastrointestinal clinics may have psychiatric disorders – mostly anxiety and depression – which might benefit by treatment. They also suggest some simple questions which are likely to help in the preliminary identification of such patients.

For anxiety:

○ Do you find you ever get anxious or frightened for no good reason?

○ Do you worry a lot about things?

For depression

○ Have you had difficulty sleeping recently?

○ Do you have spells of feeling sad or miserable?

○ Do you sometimes feel hopeless?

Not really too difficult.

Conclusion

The only safe conclusion appears to be almost wholly negative: that no final conclusion is yet possible. Of course psychological and emotional factors play a part in the syndrome. Everyone's everyday experience is enough to remind us that gut and brain are intimately linked in normal healthy individuals. So it would be odd indeed if that link was of no consequence when there's a manifest failure of some kind in the smooth running of the bowel.

This chapter has said nothing of how the brain-gut link might operate; its sole concern has been with the existence of such links. The possible nature and mechanism of these is a topic to be covered later, in Chapter 10.

If I seem to have explored this particular issue at undue length, it's because I believe it's worth trying to get at the truth, however elusive it may be. In a world free of ignorance and historical prejudice, it would matter little if this or that patient was told that his or her problem was the consequence of a neurotic predisposition, a tendency towards hysteria, or any of the rest of the lexicon of psychiatric labels which can and do in the real world give offence and cause distress. If the irritable bowel syndrome really was a consequence exclusively of one of these problems, sufferers ought to think no worse of themselves as a consequence. In reality, of course, they may well be unable to prevent themselves from doing so. Old prejudices die hard. And the attitudes of others have to be reckoned with. Neurosis is still regarded by many people as a form of moral weakness. However, as the evidence to suggest that the IBS is, of its nature, a neurotic disorder remains so equivocal, this is one burden – whether real or imagined – which sufferers shouldn't have to wrestle with.

There are, too, practical issues at stake. Leaving anxiety and depression untreated may impair the effectiveness of therapies directed specifically at the irritable bowel itself. And if patients do have untreated psychiatric as well as gut symptoms, they may find themselves returning again and again to the gastroenterological clinic for no very good purpose. The doctors who work there will grow increasingly frustrated, and perhaps decreasingly sympathetic to such patients – who might in some cases be better off seeing a specialist from the other end of the mind-body link: that is, a psychiatrist.

5 The Patients . . .
   Speaking for Themselves

He is of age; ask him:
he shall speak for himself.

St John's Gospel, 9:21

Talk to a doctor, or to any other health professional, and
you get one view of what it must be like to suffer from
this or that disorder. Talk to the patients themselves
and you often get quite another – or, in the case of the
irritable bowel syndrome, many other views. Different
people experience the disorder in different ways. Symptoms of the IBS which, to some, seem relatively trivial
are, to others, the greatest source of distress. A consultant
physician who works at the University Hospital of South
Manchester, Dr Peter Whorwell, has tried to find out how
one hundred of his IBS patients rate the relative importance of their various symptoms. He did this because he
had begun to form an impression that although a diagnosis
of the irritable bowel syndrome depends on the patient
having abdominal pain and distension, and disordered
bowel habit, many of his patients were actually more
troubled by what he calls their 'non-colonic' symptoms.

To test this suspicion he presented his patients with

a series of cards, each denoting one of these non-colonic symptoms. The patients' first task was to pick those cards identifying the symptoms from which they themselves suffered. They then had to arrange the cards they'd selected in order of importance – the most troubling symptom at the top, the least at the bottom. The first thing which Dr Whorwell discovered was that fewer than six out of every ten patients rated abdominal pain or distension or abnormal bowel habit as their most troubling symptoms. So although these are the things which define the condition, they are not necessarily the features which patients find the hardest to bear. (As Dr Whorwell points out, this may be one reason why it's so difficult to demonstrate the benefits of remedies for the IBS. If doctors define treatment success by one set of criteria, and patients by another, it's hardly surprising that clinical trials sometimes produce conflicting results. Similar confusion would arise in trying to mark a school examination if the examiners had failed to agree among themselves on the qualities they were looking for in the candidates' work.)

The non-colonic symptoms reported by the patients were (in descending order of the number of patients complaining of them) lethargy, backache, feelings of early satiety, excess wind, nausea and headache. No fewer than 96 of the 100 patients complained of lethargy.

Among the handful of patients to whom I talked, several issues came up almost every time: stress, for example. But the differences in their individual experiences, their worries, and their capacity to cope was also clear. So, following the title of the chapter, let them speak for themselves.

Patient 1: Mr G
*Mr G is thirty-four, married with two children and
head of English at a grammar school.*

I first developed the disease eleven years ago. It was
actually when I started teaching. I'm a rather tense
and nervous sort of person, though less so now than I
was then. Teaching is a very theatrical job. You're up
in front of a lot of not necessarily friendly faces who
want to be entertained and stimulated and interested.
So there is a kind of theatrical tension attached to the
job. When I started work I found I was rushing around
a lot: preparing and marking and dealing with large
numbers of often disorientated children. I became
very tense. I started getting tight knotted pains in
my stomach. One morning I found I had passed a
lot of blood. I went straight to the GP, and had it
investigated at the hospital.

At first they thought I might have colitis. I had a
barium enema, and a sigmoidoscopy and a lot of
interviews with various doctors. They couldn't find
anything physically wrong. They'd decided that it must
be the irritable bowel syndrome within about ten days
of my first going to see the GP.

The pain varies. It can be just a feeling of an
unsettled stomach, like little bubbles popping inside
my gut. At other times it can be a specific pain in
a specific place. Sometimes it's high up, and sharp
like someone pushing a knife into you; other times
it's like a knot in the abdomen. Sometimes it's just
a dull throb. I also get a feeling of expansion in the
rectum – like someone's taken a bicycle pump and
pumped me up. The pain used to double me up at
times. And the feeling of wanting to go to the loo I
found excruciating. I could put up with the pain,but
I could not put up with that. It used to drive me into

a frenzy at times. And if it occurred at work it was appalling.

They said that my smoking didn't help, so I stopped. And it did seem to relieve the symptoms. I was told that I ought to have a high fibre diet, which I dutifully followed. Initially it had some effect although I find nowadays that if I eat a lot of fibre it has the reverse effect, and makes my stomach very unsettled. So I tend not to follow that any more. I certainly couldn't eat a bowl of All-Bran now; it would choke me! I have muesli instead, which is palatable. Breakfast is very important for me. I always have a large plate of muesli, and two or three slices of wholemeal toast. I tend to eat potatoes with their jackets on. I try to avoid — although not always successfully — chocolate. I find that anything like that is bad. If I have an attack I avoid cheese as well. What suits me best is a plain, balanced diet. Rich food definitely disagrees with me, and can bring on an attack, especially garlic.

I drink much less than I used to. I'm convinced that drink has a lot to do with it — not that I'm a particularly heavy drinker. I still drink beer, but I limit it to weekends, and never have more than a couple of pints. I do find that if I have a drink every night of the week — and that's pretty rare nowadays — it seems to set the colon off, and all the symptoms recur. The only symptom which has never recurred is the bleeding.

I've been under a lot of pressure in the last few years, and I've had several attacks. I have a bad one every three months or so. But it can be more frequent than that. Working late, night after night, and missing meals — that's always fatal. If I'm not living a steady, routine sort of life it seems to trigger it.

I've largely learned how to live with the illness. When I first got it, it made me incredibly neurotic, and I would worry that it was all sorts of other things, and a vicious circle built up. Over the years I've learned to realize that this isn't a disorder I need to worry about. But I'm aware it's something I'm going to have to live with for the rest of my life. On the whole it has been much better as I've got older.

I take strenuous exercise. I run to the school every day, which is about five miles. And I swim when I get there before I start work. I do find that this helps to relax me, and that puts me in the right frame of mind to go through a day and not get uptight.

I've had to make an effort to think of myself as normal. I got myself into a state in which I thought of myself as an ill person. And that was deeply wounding to me, because I'm a very fit person. That's why I worked at trying to cope with my irritable bowel.

Not all my dealings with the doctors have been perfect. I only go to the doctor now if I develop a new symptom. The last time I went I wasn't given an examination. I said I'd had a history of the irritable bowel syndrome, but that I'd developed a new type of pain. (*It was probably proctalgia fugax (see page 175)*). The doctor said it was very common, even in people who didn't have the irritable bowel syndrome. She gave me some sedatives. And if it gets worse, she said, come back. I felt she was fobbing me off. I'd rather have had some more explanation. When it came to deciding whether or not the pain should be further investigated, she left it up to me. I felt this wasn't very helpful; after all, I'm not a doctor. I went to see the doctor for reassurance.

I must say that I have inhibitions about going to GPs over my irritable bowel. It's not that they're not interested; it's just that I feel they're not very helpful. I feel embarrassed to go because I feel I'm wasting their time. But that, I think, is partly induced by their attitude. It varies from GP to GP.

Patient 2 : Mr S
Mr S is thirty-five, single, and teaching part time while trying to find full-time work as a university lecturer.

I first started getting symptoms about four years ago, but I didn't do much about them at first. The problems I had were diarrhoea and a lot of stomach rumbling. And I felt a strange, dull, cold, hollow kind of pain when I went to the toilet. Sometimes when I went to the toilet I felt that I'd not only emptied my bowels, but passed them out as well! This worried me more than the diarrhoea, and it was this which made me go to the GP. He told me not to eat anything for a couple of days, and to come back if the diarrhoea was still troubling me. It cleared up a bit, and then it came back, and then cleared up again. But it didn't completely go away. I also had terrible wind. The outbreaks of diarrhoea didn't happen all that often – maybe about four times a year, and lasting a few days. But in the end the GP decided to refer me to the gastroenterology clinic at the hospital.

I have arthritis and psoriasis, and I thought that the bowel problems I was having were related to this. Any sort of illnesses I develop I tend to think are connected with the arthritis.

Anyway, I think my GP suspected I might have the irritable bowel syndrome, and that's why he referred me to the hospital. The consultant asked me a lot of questions to start with – about my background, my work, my eating habits, and things like that. I'm a vegetarian, and he seemed very interested in this. He wondered if I'm a fussy eater, because he said that sometimes foods can be triggers of the irritable bowel syndrome. But I don't think I'm fussy about what I eat. I only became a vegetarian because I had a girlfriend who didn't eat meat, and it was easier to eat the same sorts of things as she did.

Finally he gave me a physical examination just to check that there wasn't any sort of physical disorder in my gut. But I think he was already confident that my problem was the irritable bowel syndrome. I was with him about half an hour – which was longer than I'd expected. He gave me a prescription for dried-up seaweed or something like that (*presumably a bulking agent of some kind*). I wasn't very thrilled with that. I got it and tried it, but I didn't take it for long because I didn't like the taste. I really couldn't eat it.

I'm trying to get a job as a lecturer, and they're hard to come by. I've spent eight or ten years getting a doctorate, and qualifying for the sort of job I want. The doctor suggested that maybe it was worrying about getting a job which provoked the problem. I don't know if that's right. After all, you could say that I should have been more worried before I got my doctorate.

I got food poisoning about four or five years ago – just before I started having these gut problems. I wondered if, rather than some psychological explanation for my illness, it was this that set the problem off. I remember the occasion very well. I was working for a chain store, and I went to the staff Christmas dinner in a hotel. I got terrible food poisoning. I was alternately throwing up and sitting on the toilet and fainting. This happened four times during the morning after the meal. It was really awful. I couldn't believe that I could keep on being sick; I couldn't believe there was anything left in me after the second time of throwing up! I don't know if there is a connection between this illness and the later problems; but they did start shortly after this time. Or maybe it's a combination of this and the psychological problems, the worry about finding a job.

Patient 3 : Mrs D
Mrs D is aged thirty-nine, married, and a junior school teacher.

The first time I realized that anything was wrong was at a rather posh dinner party. My problem is what you might call a noisy one. If you can imagine what your central heating sounds like when it goes wrong – the noises in the pipes – well, my tummy makes noises like that. I was horrified when it started producing these dreadful sounds. But I thought it was a one-off. Everybody laughed, and I forgot about it.

The problem didn't really develop badly for a few more years. Now and then it played up, but it wasn't a real difficulty till about seven years ago. When I first got back to this country I was immersed in doing an Open University degree, and I didn't have much time to think about my health. All my thoughts were taken up doing the course, and by my social life which was quite full. But when I'd got my degree, which was when I was about thirty-one, I had more time on my hands. The problem then started to get much worse. As well as the noise I get the feeling that I'm full of air. I feel bloated. I find when it starts that I have to go to the loo a bit more; but the main problem is simply the noise. If it was just the rumbling sound you get when you're hungry, I could cope with it. But the noise is much much worse than that. Men can carry this sort of thing off. But it's much harder for women.

I think the problem is made worse by worrying about it. The noise tends to happen whenever it's going to be most embarrassing. I'm quite a social person, and I mix a lot. My stomach makes noises from time to time during any normal day – but then it doesn't matter. If it happens in the classroom it's of no significance either, so I don't worry about it. But I get very upset if it happens in a social venue because I like to think of myself as being fairly sophisticated.

It really has restricted my life, and I'm very upset about that. I haven't been to a theatre for six or seven years. I'll go to a musical or an opera as long as it's something fairly noisy. But you wouldn't get me sitting through a drama because I'd be so rigid with fear.

Over the years I've tried just about everything to stop it. First of all I thought it might be diet, so I went to a clinic and paid an awful lot of money. I thought it might be an allergy. They put me on what they called a 'stone-age diet'. They gradually introduced other foods, but they didn't manage to show that any particular food was causing the problem. Then they thought it might be caused by Candida, the fungus. But the treatment for this didn't really seem to do anything.

Then I went to a natural health clinic. They gave me lots of different vitamins. But this didn't work. When you're desperate you'll try anything that might offer hope. I also had hypnosis. That seemed to help a little.

In teaching now we have a lot of meetings. I find it very difficult professionally because I dread sitting in a quiet room or a lecture theatre. So I tend to avoid any sort of courses, which isn't doing me any good professionally. I haven't gone for promotion which I would have done otherwise.

The first GP I had was very good. He knew how to handle me. He was very reassuring. And that seemed to stop me worrying, and the problem didn't happen so often. But then things got worse, and I went to a different GP. His attitude was, 'Hard luck. You're not going to die of it. You'll just have to pull yourself together and face up to it.'

I do now have various things which help. Tranquillizers seem to make a difference, so I take one if I've got something stressful ahead of me – a staff meeting or a dinner party or something like that. Also a private doctor I went to told me take Imodium (*loperamide, a drug which acts on the muscles of the gut wall, and is used to treat diarrhoea*). I have to take it the day before an event which might be worrying me. I really do feel it works – but it isn't ideal. After taking it, I need a few days to get back to normal. So I can't take it every day. I have restricted it to occasions which are likely to be most traumatic or to create problems.

Another thing which helps a bit is alcohol. Two or three drinks, either wine or brandy, make me a lot better. Maybe it's some direct effect on the gut, or perhaps it simply relaxes me. I stop worrying about the problem, and this in itself makes the noises less likely to happen. I've been referred to gastroenterologists, but I've just been laughed out of the room. Because it's not going to kill you, they don't necessarily take it very seriously. One I saw said, 'We've got a nurse here with the same problem. You just have to laugh when it happens.' You feel so small when they say things like that. And I suppose it's true that there are other people around hospital with far worse things – diseases which might actually kill them. So on the one hand I feel guilty about making a fuss about it; but on the other hand it does make me very unhappy, and it affects my life very much. It's not very nice being laughed at because of something you can't control.

It's not the sort of thing you can talk about, except with very close friends. When I'm with friends I ask them if we can have music on in the background. When I'm asked out to dinner I always say, 'Don't forget about the music!' I'm always entertaining here, at home, because I'm in charge, and I can make sure the music's on loud enough.

I didn't think that I would ever get married. When the problem started to get bad, it cramped my style enormously. In fact I met someone who's incredibly kind. It doesn't matter to him at all. But before I met him it was very difficult. With each person I had to decide whether or not to say anything. I felt I'd be a social burden. At one stage I started to avoid physical relationships. I thought the stomach noises would put anyone off. After making love I used to say something like, 'I'm not very good at sleeping in the same bed with anyone else, so do you mind using the bed in the spare room?' I couldn't bear the thought of lying there with someone and having my stomach start making its noises. I really felt I'd rather spend my life on my own.

I'm locked into a vicious circle; the more I don't want it to happen, the more likely it is to happen. The only thing I can compare it to is stuttering, where the stutter starts when it's most important not to stutter. You feel beaten by it; you feel it will always get you when it matters.

I'm now seeing a psychologist at the hospital, and he's teaching me relaxation. But I'm not at all certain it will work; it's very difficult to surmount your gut! It's a formidable rival.

Patient 4 : Ms H
Ms H is a beautician who runs her own business. She's twenty-four and single.

I've always had problems with my stomach, either diarrhoea or constipation. I'd have trouble after Indian or any other spicy food. But about a year ago I started being under a lot of stress, and the problem got much worse. I had a lot of work problems, and I also got very fed up with myself. I wanted to change this and I wanted to change that. Perhaps it was frustration more than stress. At that time I started eating a lot of junk food, never sitting down to a proper meal or taking time over eating. I think that aggravated the gut problems.

I couldn't eat anything without having to go to the toilet very often. It wasn't just spicy food that upset me. I cut out cheese and all other dairy products, and all red meat; I had no fried or fatty stuff. All I was eating was fish and poultry. Yet I couldn't leave home in the morning before I'd gone to the toilet about four times. The diet didn't solve the problem – but at least it helped me to lose a lot of weight!

My stomach felt very bloated all the time; in fact I looked as if I might be pregnant. This was very embarrassing; it doesn't look good if a beauty therapist can't control her own weight and appearance! I also had a lot of pain in the lower right part of my abdomen. It was a sharp pain which surged to a peak for a few seconds, and then went away. I used to get giddy and feel as if I was going to pass out. This would happen at various times during the day. I tried all the usual upset stomach remedies, and things like kaolin and morphine. This went on for a few months before I decided it was time to go to the doctor.

The GP was really good. I'd had my appendix out some while ago, and he thought my problem might be caused by adhesions. Actually it was me who suggested it might be the irritable bowel syndrome! I have a habit of going through medical encyclopaedias when something's wrong with me. So I thought it was either an ulcer or an irritable bowel.

I hadn't thought of adhesions. I didn't think it was cancer.

The GP referred me to the hospital specialist. He asked me a lot of questions and gave me an internal examination. He said it was almost certainly an irritable bowel, and if I wanted to get rid of it I'd have to change my lifestyle. He prescribed a binding agent of some kind. It was very reassuring to know what the problem was. It can be quite worrying if you don't know what's causing the problem.

Right now the problem's almost cleared up. But it does come on again if I'm under stress. Because my company is very small, if I have a bad week it shows in the bank balance very sharply. That's when the bowel problem starts again. I think I'm always going to get it because I'm a worrier.

My advice to anyone with the irritable bowel syndrome is to analyse their life, emotional and physical, to find out what's triggering the problem. For me it's stress – so I think that's the first thing to look at. If you can anticipate when you're going to be put under pressure, you stand a chance of being able to transform that pressure into a minor irritation. Then start looking at the food you eat. But I'd say look at your mental wellbeing first, because that seems to be responsible for so much of the problem.

Patient 5 : Ms T
Ms T is single, thirty-two and works as a studio sound technician.

I've had the irritable bowel syndrome twice. The first time it came I was about twenty-one and taking my degree. It lasted for about a year. Then there was a gap of eight or nine years before it started again. I was then about thirty. And that time too it lasted about a year. I'm now through it; but the symptoms do recur from time to time.

The first time round I had more stomach problems than bowel problems. I had a lot of abdominal pain, difficulties with digestion – wind and belching – and sometimes constipation for several days. The second time it was quite different. I had the wind, the belching, and the abdominal pain that I'd had before; but instead of constipation I had a lot of diarrhoea – which was very upsetting and embarrassing and inconvenient.

The problem was with me most of the time. There might be a few days when everything settled down to normal; but then the symptoms would come back exactly as before. And with them would come feelings of depression: I'm in a prison, this is something I'm never going to be able to get rid of, why me?

I tried a lot of things to stop the symptoms. I altered my diet. For example I eliminated all wheat products and dairy foods. I had soya milk instead. I tried a lot of the obvious medicines like kaolin and morphine for the diarrhoea. I also tried relaxation. I went to a clinical psychologist. I tried to examine my own nature to see if I could control what I was doing. I tried more exercise, I tried changing my social patterns, I cut out drink for a while, I tried to rest more. But none of these things were very effective.

I think the whole thing is to do with stress. The first time I was very worried about my examinations and about getting my degree. The second time it was an emotional involvement which was causing conflicting feelings within myself. Although I was experiencing moments of great happiness, there were also times of enormous depression. Both times the problems cleared up when the things which were worrying me solved themselves.

The first time round I went to the GP after about two or three months. He thought it was a question of stomach acid, and he gave me treatment for that. That didn't make much difference. And as I hadn't wanted to take tablets in the first place, it actually made me feel even worse. He also sent me for a barium meal, presumably to make sure I hadn't got an ulcer. But of course that turned out negative.

The second time I tolerated the symptoms for more like four or five months. The GP didn't take the problem very seriously; but I did eventually get to see a specialist. I took along a detailed list of everything which had gone on, and he said he thought it was the irritable bowel syndrome. He then did an examination, and couldn't find anything physically the matter. He referred me to a clinical psychologist. It's always nice to talk to understanding people, but I'm not sure it did very much good.

The constant worry of the irritable bowel syndrome is very fatiguing, and depressing. It's a burden you carry around because you feel slightly unclean. If something else creates serious emotional problems in my life, I suspect the whole thing will start again.

Patient 6 : Ms M
Ms M is thirty-three, single, and a lecturer.

I began having problems about two years ago. I'd had a very bad bout of 'flu and I didn't recover from that. I more or less collapsed with what must have been the post-viral fatigue syndrome. I couldn't concentrate on anything; I couldn't work; I couldn't watch television; I slept almost all the time. I was totally exhausted. It was

when I was coming out of that that I started having
digestive problems.

My main problem was going from a week or so
of constipation through to diarrhoea for a few days,
and then back to constipation. And terrible pain and
flatulence, especially after my evening meal. Even in
my normal state I err on the side of constipation.

I took Milk of Magnesia, Alka-Seltzer and other
home remedies like that. I cut out all fizzy drinks
because these made my abdomen extremely painful.
After a few weeks I went to the GP. She was very
sympathetic, very thorough, and never dismissive. She
suspected it might be the irritable bowel syndrome.
She prescribed Colpermin [peppermint oil], and
Regulan [ispaghula husk]. The Colpermin definitely
helped. I was supposed to take two sachets of
Regulan each day, but it gave me far too much
flatulence. Increasing the fibre in my diet also
increases the pain and flatulence.

The GP referred me to the specialist, and he
gave me a barium enema. He said, 'This problem
is just something you young women have', and then
dismissed me. He was totally patronizing about it.

I now know that certain things don't agree with me.
Weetabix, coffee, cider and so on. I love stir-fried
vegetables, but I can't eat them. My evening meal's
the main problem. I can still get very bloated, and then
have a lot of flatulence.

At one point I tried a simplified diet which had
helped a friend of mine. It consisted of roast chicken,
rice, green vegetables, fresh fruit, and bottled water.
But it made me extremely ill. After two weeks I
stopped the chicken and had fish instead. But I was
still ill so I packed it up. I'd recently had an attack of
gastroenteritis, so maybe it was something to do with
that. That's what the doctor thought, anyway.

I think that stress had something to do with the
whole thing. The four months before I had the original

'flu was a period of great stress for me. I was having terrible problems with my PhD thesis, and I was also having other work problems. Perhaps stress set off the post-viral problems, *and* the irritable bowel syndrome.

I now feel I know how best to cope with my bowels. I won't be having any more hospital appointments unless it gets worse, or I have any new symptoms. But I still have problems. For some reason I had terrible problems – a pain and wind – today when I was in Sainsbury's. It's fortunate that the store has a toilet!

Patient 7: Mrs K
Mrs K is forty-seven, and married with two children. She lectures in social studies.

The symptoms first appeared about twelve years ago. They came completely out of the blue when I was driving back from a business lunch. It was like a migraine accompanied by a strong spasm in the abdomen, and a sudden urge to vomit. After this I had something of the kind about once every three months. The vomiting is awful; and it can go on all day. I didn't go to the doctor because I was sure it was all brought on by stress. The problem did seem to occur on those occasions when I had to perform well at work.

Some time after that I started to develop a lot of pain in the abdomen, and difficulties with my bowels – back and forth between constipation and diarrhoea. I felt a real malaise. I also got a very dry mouth, and sore lips. An attack could be very debilitating; it would knock me out for a few days. I got very alarmed, so I went to the GP who referred me to a gastroenterologist. I had a barium meal and a few other tests, and they said I had a spastic colon. They said it was likely to cause problems from time to time, and there wasn't much they could do. They said I'd just have to steer clear of processed foods, and eat lots of bran.

I changed my diet and did eat a lot of whole foods. It seemed to help a bit. But the main thing was that I was relieved to hear that I didn't have some ghastly growth. I learned to live with the symptoms, and not get very frightened. Things seemed to stabilize after this, especially for the next couple of years while I was living in France. I'm sure the change of diet made a lot of difference.

When I came back to Britain the problem started to get worse. I went to the GP again – a different one this time. He said it was the irritable bowel syndrome, and he put me on to drug treatment: a combination of Cimetidine *[an anti-ulcer drug]*, and also a combination of a tranquillizer and an anti-spasmodic. Unfortunately this is no longer available, and nothing else seems to work so well. While I was taking this things weren't too bad.

Over the last two years it's got a lot worse. I've been going through the menopause, and I remarried. I'm sure that both these things have played a part in setting the problem off again. Now I don't use any treatment. Clearly the whole thing is stress related, and I've got to live with it.

Most of the doctors I've seen – apart from one GP – haven't been much help. I've had the feeling they just want me out of the door as soon as possible.

6 Dietary Treatments

Give me neither poverty nor riches;
feed me with food convenient for me.

Proverbs 30: 8

The gut's most regular, most enduring, and most variable experience of the outside world is the food which we choose to inflict upon it. Ignoring dietary change as a possible way of tackling the irritable bowel syndrome would be like refusing to contemplate a splint for a broken leg. You don't have to believe that diet is at the root of the disorder to wonder if changing what is eaten might have some beneficial effect. Headaches aren't caused by an insufficiency of aspirin; but aspirin may overcome them.

At the top of the menu, of course, is fibre. Like many dietary constituents, fibre has long been prey to changing ideas – and sometimes changing fashion. There was a time when most patients with bowel disturbances were recommended to eat a diet low in fibre on the grounds that having a large quantity of undigestible material in the gut could serve only to irritate it. A low fibre diet was thought to allow the bowel's tired and irritable muscles an opportunity for rest and relaxation. Having too much material in the large bowel was also claimed to bring about 'autointoxication'. This rather mysterious condition was supposed to be characterized by all sorts of symptoms including headache, halitosis (bad breath), flatulence, premature senility, falling hair, depression and insomnia. Its champions claimed that toxins (never identified) absorbed from the large bowel poisoned the body. So wholeheartedly did some of them believe in this theory that they suggested we should all have our large bowels surgically removed!

The next best thing to having no colon was thought to be speeding material through it as rapidly as possible. This, of course, involved eating foods with a high fibre content. Some of the doctors who viewed the colon with such mistrust were thus advocating what we nowadays regard as a good diet – though they were doing so for the wrong reasons. Bowel habits and all processes associated with them have seldom, for some reason, prompted clear and rational thought. Prejudice and superstition have always flourished in the gut.

As already explained, the renewed interest in fibre originated with a handful of doctors, whose experience of studying illness in various far-flung parts of the world led them to believe (on the basis of extremely slim evidence) that a shortage of fibre is responsible for a range of sickness, from heart disease to cancer. The effect of fibre on the irritable bowel syndrome has since been investigated by a number of research groups, but not all these studies have reached quite the same conclusion.

The resurgence of enthusiasm for bran hit Britain during the 1970s. Dr Ken Heaton of Bristol University, one of the country's leading authorities on dietary fibre and its effects, believes that several findings accounted for this *volte face*. One of them, ironically, was a small and uncontrolled trial of bran in which twenty-three out of thirty IBS patients taking it reported relief of their symptoms. At the time of this report (1974) it was not generally realized how powerful the placebo effect can be in helping IBS patients. (The placebo effect is the improvement that some patients will experience following a treatment simply because they expect that treatment to help them.) But as Dr Heaton has pointed out, 'Doctors were ready for a new approach to treatment, and not disposed to be unduly sceptical.'

Drs Ken Heaton and Richard Harvey have come up with some of the more encouraging evidence about the benefits of fibre. Towards the end of the 1970s, they compared the progress of a group of IBS patients eating a diet in wheat fibre with another eating a low fibre diet. Patients in the former group took their extra fibre in the form of unprocessed wheat bran (a little under an ounce), or brown bread (four standard slices), or a combination of both. Bran is not the most appetizing food in the world, and patients weren't expected to eat their daily dose in one sitting. Their counterparts eating a low fibre diet had to keep off all wholegrain cereal products, and to limit their intake of fruit and vegetables. Both groups of patients were asked to keep to their respective diets for six weeks. At the end of each day they used special charts to record the stools they had passed, and any pain they had felt.

Before the experiment began, one of the researchers had interviewed all the subjects to obtain full details of their symptoms. Subjects also had to agree to measurements being made of the muscular activity going on within their large bowels. This was much to their credit as it involved spending an hour with a small pressure-measuring balloon inserted through the anus! At the end of the six weeks the researchers repeated both the questioning and measurements.

By the end of the study, the high fibre diet group were on the whole suffering less pain less often, and had a more satisfactory bowel habit. The balloon measurements revealed that the high fibre diet was also associated with a reduced level of activity within the large bowel. The bran seemed not to do any better than the wholewheat bread – which is fortunate because, as the Bristol doctors rightly pointed out, this is a more pleasant way of taking the required quantity of fibre.

Alas, nothing about the irritable bowel syndrome is straightforward, and this encouraging picture is slightly muddied by the work of four New Zealand doctors who reported their findings in 1984. Like the Bristol group, they rated their patients' pain and other symptoms before and after putting them on a high fibre diet. Instead of specifying an exact quantity of fibre to be eaten, they gave the patients a booklet explaining which foods are rich in it. The booklet also contained sample recipes. They checked their patients' actual increase in fibre consumption by measuring the quantity and type of the food being eaten, and by weighing each subject's stools.

It turned out that the diets eaten by the patients increased their fibre intakes by about the same amount as that specified in the Bristol experiments. And the symptoms of about half the patients improved greatly following the switch to a high fibre diet. But, two or three years later, when the researchers followed up their subjects' progress, the extent of the improvement bore little relation to individual increases in fibre intake. It's not entirely clear what we should make of this finding. The researchers themselves take it to mean that while fibre may be useful in relieving specific symptoms such as constipation, it shouldn't be seen as a panacea: something which solves all problems. They say it should be part of a total management plan in which patient support and reassurance are also important. And that, surely, is indisputable.

It's worth remembering that not everyone responds well

to increased levels of fibre, and that it actually makes some patients' symptoms worse. Some people find bran too unpalatable. Such individuals may get on better with an artificial bulking agent. The commonest is psyllium or ispaghula husk, a material derived from the seeds of an Indian plant. This has a high water-holding capacity, and creates a more substantial stool. Commercial preparations (Metamucil, Fybogel, and so on) come as unappetizing dry powders or flaky granules which are best taken dispersed in water or some other drink. The ideal dose – usually of the order of a tablespoonful at least twice a day – can be judged on the basis of experience.

Reviewing the evidence on fibre

In the mid 1980s Dr Heaton looked through all the published studies of the value of dietary fibre, and commented that when you consider how common the IBS is, surprisingly few attempts had been made to evaluate the effects of fibre. At that time there were just three full reports on bran, together with two more studies published only in outline. There were also two trials of ispaghula. For reasons which can only be guessed at, two of the five full reports showed bran to have a significantly beneficial effect, while the remaining three did not. In an effort to pull in further relevant data, and make a more rounded picture, Dr Heaton decided to review the effects of controlled trials of bran on patients with diverticular disease. A diverticulum is a pouch which forms at a weak point in the wall of the gut. Diverticular disease is a consequence of the formation of these pouches in the colon, and is often associated with pain in the abdomen and disturbances of bowel habit. This is another condition in which bran has become a standard treatment. But here too there was conflict, because two trials came out in favour of bran, while another did not.

Understandably, Dr Heaton's only definite conclusion was that no definite conclusion would be possible until more, and more carefully designed, studies had been carried out. The only things which emerged unequivocally were that the placebo effect of treatment can be considerable (it rose to an extraordinary 71 per cent in one study) and that bran is most likely to be effective in constipated patients. In so far as any treatment can be conducted rationally under these difficult circumstances, Dr Heaton starts by recommending wholemeal bread and other foods rich in fibre; he waits to see how well these work before going on to suggest bran, or to prescribe other bulking agents. Raw bran has the obvious advantage of being cheap, but not all patients tolerate it well. Cooked bran of the type found in breakfast cereal is the next best thing.

Despite the lack of definitive proof, many (perhaps most) doctors now believe that a high fibre diet is worth trying. The balance of the evidence is that it shortens the time required for food to make its passage through the body, and benefits patients with both constipation and diarrhoea. It's also simple (a spoonful of bran per meal), and has relatively few side effects (except for an initial increase in gas) – both of which are more than can be said for many treatments nowadays. In short, well worth a try.

Example of a high fibre diet

Breakfast
Orange juice or half grapefruit.
Muesli, oatmeal porridge or bran cereal.
Wholemeal bread or toast, oatcakes or crispbread.
Coarse-cut marmalade.

Lunch

Vegetable soup, including chopped fresh vegetables,
lentils, barley, etc.
Sandwiches (wholemeal bread) filled with salad,
and including celery or grated carrots.

Tea

Wholemeal wheat biscuits, oatcakes or crispbread.

Dinner

Meat or fish.
Potato baked in its jacket.
Green beans.
Salad.
Wholemeal bread.
Fruit.

Tea and coffee may be drunk with all meals.

Food intolerance

At present, if your GP refers you to a gastroenterologist on
account of the irritable bowel syndrome, it's unlikely that
you will be tested for food intolerance, never mind treated
for it. The reasons are good and bad. The good reason
might be that the doctor you are seeing has familiarized
himself with the evidence, and judged either that it's not
persuasive, or that his particular clinic doesn't have the
resources or the time or the staff to organize the fairly
elaborate process of identifying a troublesome food. The

bad reason would be that too many doctors still don't take food very seriously.

The teaching on food and nutrition was still quite primitive when many of today's doctors qualified. They may well have learned the classic stuff; how scurvy results from lack of vitamin C, and how the far-sighted British navy prevented it by carrying lime juice on all its ships. But many of the more recent insights are less straightforward, and much less dramatic than the effects of insufficient vitamin C. To make matters worse, the field of food intolerance-cum-allergy is bedevilled by self-appointed experts who are at best confused about the topic, at worst charlatans. Unwilling to dabble in something so often associated with the fringe, some doctors prefer simply to neglect it altogether.

In principle there's nothing to stop the IBS sufferer organizing his or her own exclusion diet, and staged reintroduction of individual foods. But a couple of caveats. Never rely on your own diagnosis. Be sure that the IBS really is what you're suffering from before you take a self-help path. And even when you have decided to try it for yourself, you'll need the co-operation of other members of the family, and a great deal of willpower. If you're not naturally a systematic, organized kind of person, you must accept that your life is going to have to change radically for the three or four months it may take to reach the answers you want.

You can find an outline of what's involved in this approach in the food intolerance section on page 43. Dr Hunter offers a number of practical tips. The exclusion diet itself comprises meat (but not bacon, sausages, or anything else which may contain preservatives); white fish (but not smoked or shell fish); vegetables except for potatoes, onions and sweetcorn; non-citrus fruit; rice products (not wheat); olive, soya and sunflower oil but not corn or vegetable oil; goat, sheep and soya milk and their derivatives, but no other dairy products; and herbal teas and non-citrus fruit juices. An exclusion diet, even if it *is* going to work, may not show any evidence of benefit for the first seven days; so the second week will require extra perseverance. Try to eat as many as possible of the allowed foods; a few even of these do affect some people. If the list includes any which you already suspect might be causing you a problem, leave them out too.

If your condition really has improved at the end of the two weeks, reintroduce the foods one at a time for two days each in a set order. Keep a diary of how you feel; this will help you to notice if any of the foods are provoking IBS symptoms. Eat plenty of each food. If you have any doubts about a particular food, don't spend too long on trying it out. Leave it out and come back to it later. Finally, retest the suspect foods to make sure that you really have identified the ones which are causing problems. If you find that the list of foods you can't take has grown too long, you may have to abandon this approach to the IBS as impractical. If you still wish to press on, get the advice of a dietician to make sure that you are not going to suffer from malnourishment.

You can find full details of this approach to the irritable bowel – plus a selection of recipes – in a book called *The Allergy Diet*. It's published by Martin Dunitz/Macdonald Optima, and its authors are Dr John Hunter, Elizabeth Workman and Dr Virginia Alun Jones. To make a success of discovering a food intolerance problem, and then to solve it by your own efforts, you really do need this book or something like it. It would be a shame to spoil the attempt for the lack of a few practical hints.

7   Drug Treatments

The desire to take medicine is perhaps
the greatest feature which distinguishes
man from animals.

Sir William Osler

Rich industrial societies like our own have, in recent
years, developed extraordinarily ambivalent if not contradictory attitudes towards medicinal drugs. Some of us feel
cheated if the GP doesn't round off the consultation with
a prescription to be taken to the chemist. 'A pill for every
ill' is the unspoken assumption here. All animals sleep,
breathe, look for food, and choose a mate; many build
shelters; some play, at least when young. But as the
physician Sir William Osler noted, only humans take
medicines. Indeed, it has been such a feature of most
human societies at most times that it might almost
be regarded as one of the defining characteristics of
our species. There have, though, always been people
who deplore the enthusiasm for medication. Witness the
words of the American Oliver Wendell Holmes writing
more than a century ago: 'If the whole of the materia
medica ... could be sunk to the bottom of the sea, it

would be all the better for mankind, and all the worse for the fishes.'

It was the Thalidomide tragedy of the early sixties which transformed unease into outright hostility: an antagonism directed to some extent against the drugs themselves, but even more towards the industry which invents, makes and sells them. Two comments are worth bearing in mind. The first is that there can be no such thing as a drug without side effects. To borrow the pithy words of the first chairman of what is now the Committee on Safety of Medicines, show me a drug without side effects, and I'll show you a drug which does nothing. The second thing to remember is that medicines are more intensively tested and more tightly regulated than almost any other commercial product, with the possible exception of civil aircraft. This is not to suggest that no future drug will bring about a re-run of the Thalidomide affair. All that can be said with conviction is that the present drug regulations have vastly reduced the likelihood of such an episode.

One of the pitfalls of any attempt to judge the usefulness of a drug is the placebo response (see page 118). The irritable bowel syndrome is no exception to this rule, and its very nature makes the assessment of benefit still more hazardous, because the various symptoms of the collection which go to make up the IBS seem to have different likelihoods of responding to a placebo. According to one assessment, diarrhoea and feelings of distension normally show a placebo response rate of about 30 per cent; in other words, roughly three out of every ten patients with those symptoms will report some improvement even when, unknowingly, the treatment they have been taking consists of dummy pills. On the other hand constipation and pain, under the very same circumstances, may show a 50 per cent placebo response. Pity the wretched researcher contemplating his data and trying to decide if he has made a valuable breakthrough, or if his experiments have really proved absolutely nothing!

On then to specifics: the drugs which doctors might prescribe for the irritable bowel syndrome. Most of them fall into two categories: antispasmodics to relieve the pain and discomfort, and psychoactive drugs.

Antispasmodics

An antispasmodic drug does more or less what its name suggests: it causes muscles to relax. The muscles which ring the gut and variously squeeze, stir and propel its contents onward are of a type known as 'smooth'. Smooth muscle is also found in other systems of the body including the blood vessels, the airways, and the bladder. All muscles receive their controlling instructions in the form of nerve impulses. Different types of muscle are under the control of different branches of the nervous system. Smooth muscles receive their instructions from the autonomic system.

To understand how the drugs used to make these muscles relax actually work, you have first to understand what goes on when the brain transmits a message to the gut. The message itself travels in the form of a series of electrical impulses via the nerve which runs to the particular group of muscles which the brain wants to influence. Once the message has reached the muscle fibres, it's again conducted along them electrically. But somehow the message has to jump the gap – a small one, but a gap nonetheless – separating the end of the nerve from the surface of the muscle fibre it's supposed to communicate with. This narrow space is bridged not electrically, but chemically.

The arrival of the electrical impulse at the end of the nerve causes it to pump out a tiny quantity of a specific chemical. This diffuses across to the far side of the gap where some of it will impinge on special sites on the surface of the muscle called receptors. If you think of these as locked switches, the molecules of the chemical messenger released by the nerve ending are able to act as the key. Only a molecule of the right shape will fit on to the receptor; when it does so, it unlocks the switch, and turns it on. It's this which sets off the electrical impulse in the muscle – and so causes it to contract. An enzyme then destroys the chemical messenger, and the receptor switches itself off until the next molecule arrives.

Different types of nerve and muscle use different chemicals to transmit their messages. The parasympathetic nerves – the ones which make the gut muscles contract and generally keep it active – use a chemical called acetylcholine. If follows that anything you do to interfere with the ability of the nerves to make acetylcholine, or to destroy the acetylcholine which has been made, or to prevent the muscle's receptors from responding to acetylcholine, will effectively disrupt the message system. The brain can send as many messages as it likes to the gut, telling it to contract more vigorously; but if those messages aren't able to make it across the gap separating the nerve endings from the gut's muscles, those muscles won't respond.

That, at any rate, is the theory. The practice is a little less impressive. The drugs – there are many of them – which have this effect of disrupting the acetylcholine message system are known as 'anticholinergics'. Despite being commonly prescribed, the evidence that they do precisely what they're supposed to do is a shade less than substantial. A great deal of the research on their medical value seems to be fatally flawed – a not uncommon state of affairs when people who may be very good doctors turn their hand to science. Some doctors make first-rate scientists, designing their investigations in such a way as to avoid ambiguity and ensure that the results, whatever they are, actually reveal something. Others – through arrogance, ignorance, desperation for career reasons to have something published, or simple carelessness – design investigations which of their nature (being too small, with no controls, with poorly diagnosed subjects, and so on) can reveal nothing. The literature of 'scientific' medicine is awash with such reports.

But enough of hobbyhorses. One doctor who has ploughed through the published reports of his fellow professionals concludes that there is some suggestion that anticholinergic drugs help patients whose main symptom is pain and/or constipation. But there is no convincing evidence, either theoretical or experimental, that these drugs are good for patients whose main symptom is diarrhoea.

And then, of course, there is the matter of side effects. Anticholinergic drugs have an effect on all systems of the body in which acetycholine has a part to play – and there are many such systems. For example, they cause a dry mouth, reduced sweating, increased heart rate, blurred vision, dilated pupils and restlessness. The greater the dose, the more likely is the taker to suffer any or all of these. In moderate doses, none of these side effects may prove to be a problem. And as with all drugs, side effects are a variable phenomenon; of two people taking identical drugs in identical amounts, only one may experience them. The aim in drug therapy is to find a balance between the effects which you want, and those which you don't: a therapeutic happy medium.

A study reported a few years ago showed that peppermint oil is a good treatment for the irritable bowel syndrome. Peppermint oil is a naturally occurring material known for its anti-flatulence properties. It seems to work by relaxing the smooth muscle of the gut. Some doctors in Manchester and Wales carried out a controlled trial in which half of a group of patients were given capsules of oil packaged in such a way that their contents would not be released until they had passed through the stomach and into the part of the gut where their effects were needed. Another group of patients took dummy capsules. For the next three weeks, all the patients graded their symptoms daily on a five-point scale. The peppermint oil group experienced more improvement in their symptoms than did the group taking the dummy capsules. But it's difficult to know what to make of this and similar such studies. How many doctors are actually using peppermint oil for these purposes is anyone's guess.

Psychoactive drugs

Psychoactive drugs are the second broad category used for treating IBS patients. The word 'psychoactive' is simply a term used to describe any drug which affects the taker's mood and behaviour. There is no very good evidence that these drugs affect the bowel itself. What they can do is influence the taker's state of mind. If you hold to the view that the IBS is primarily a consequence of what's going on in the sufferer's head, the logic of using a psychoactive drug is clear enough. But you don't have to take this view to justify the use of these drugs. Even if all the anxiety and depression which accompany the syndrome are a consequence and not a cause of the IBS, they still merit treatment. For one thing it's unkind to leave patients in a state of mental distress without doing something about it; for another, leaving the anxiety and depression untreated could delay or otherwise hinder the treatment of whatever malfunction really is at the core of the IBS.

Drugs intended to treat anxiety are called anxiolytics or minor tranquillizers. The agents most commonly used belong to a group of chemicals called the benzodiazepines, the best known member of which is Valium. Their main effect is to calm you down – and, in larger doses, send you to sleep. Not surprisingly, one of their adverse effects when taken in even small doses is drowsiness. They can also cause feelings of light-headedness and lack of co-ordination – symptoms which may persist into the day following that on which they were taken. In recent years there has been much concern about the addictive proper-ties of the benzodiazepines. Originally, such suggestions were disputed. Now there is a general acceptance that regular and prolonged use can lead to dependency.

People who've become dependent on a drug and then stop taking it suffer withdrawal symptoms. These include nausea, sweating, palpitations, insomnia, severe anxiety and, in extreme cases, hallucinations. The way to avoid dependence is to take as small a dose as possible for as short a time as possible. There is no need to be frightened of these drugs provided you use them sensibly. It's worth remembering, incidentally, that when benzodiazepines are used for long periods they become progressively less effective at dealing with the problem for which they were originally prescribed. So besides the dangers of addiction, it's pointless to go on and on taking them. Unfortunately, the irritable bowel syndrome itself can go on and on. So to get the most benefit from these drugs, you should only take Valium or its equivalents when things are particu-larly tough.

Anti-depressant drugs do precisely what their name suggests. There are many different varieties, each – if the pharmaceutical industry is to be believed – with its own special set of advantages. Most doctors use a small selection which they have got to know well. Different members of the anti-depressant group have different side effects, many of them not unlike those already listed for the anti-anxiety drugs. But by contrast, none of the anti-depressants commonly in use seems to produce dependence.

Because the irritable bowel syndrome comprises a spectrum of symptoms of different relative importance in different patients, the doctor may feel the need to tackle one or more symptoms in particular. Diarrhoea, for example. The use of dietary fibre has already been described. Other ways of tackling it include kaolin, codeine, various newer drugs such as loperamide, and an unpalatable powdery form of resin called cholestyramine.

All manner of combinations of drug types have been tried at different times by different physicians. One favoured combination is bran or some artificial bulking agent plus a psychoactive drug plus an anti-spasmodic. If it's difficult to assess the benefits of one drug at a time, trying to find out which of various combinations is likely to give the best results is a Herculean task. Indeed, Hercules himself would have reason to feel that merely cleaning the Augean stables was a modest challenge compared with that of deciding which of various drug combinations might most effectively have limited the capacity of the Augean horses to foul them in the first place! However, at least one doctor has tackled the enterprise and convinced himself that this triple therapy is a useful way of dealing with the IBS. Unfortunately not all his colleagues agree that the case has been made sufficiently convincingly for this type of approach to be used routinely.

All in all, drug treatment for the IBS is not one of medicine's triumphs. Reading some of the medical literature about the value and appropriate use of drugs in this field is a dispiriting experience. Much of the careful experimental evaluation which needs to be done hasn't been done. In part, this is because of the difficulty of precisely categorizing the patients being treated. In part, too, it's that recurring feature of the irritable bowel syndrome: its sheer complexity. Indeed, given the interplay of factors which seem to account for the IBS, one reviewer has remarked rather gloomily that 'no drug can be expected to have a lasting, broad-spectrum effect'. Perhaps that's too pessimistic. Either way, doctors being – like the rest of us –

creatures of habit, they tend to adopt certain patterns of drug prescribing, and then stick to them even when the evidence that they do much good isn't forthcoming. But that's not to imply that drug treatments are pointless. Some do work for some people.

8 Hypnosis

Canst thou not administer to a mind
  diseas'd
Pluck from the memory a rooted
  sorrow
Raze out the written troubles of the
  brain,
And with some sweet oblivious
  antidote
Cleanse the stuff'd bosom of that
  perilous stuff
Which weighs upon the heart?

                                    Macbeth

To some patients suffering from the irritable bowel syndrome, the thought of having it treated by hypnosis will be almost as unsettling as the illness itself. After all, we all know what hypnosis is like – or rather we think we do. A score of old films have left deep impressions of men with wild, staring eyes, sharply pointed beards, and strong Viennese accents who swing gold watch chains in front of their victims' passive, expressionless faces. A droning but impelling voice commands the subject to 'Look into my eyes . . . ' Alternatively, but no less disturbingly, there are recollections of the stage hypnotist whose subjects are commanded to behave like chickens, or to imitate chimpanzees – and all for the benefit of a voyeuristic audience. Can these shenanigans possibly have anything to do with curing an illness?

They haven't, of course; medical hypnosis bears little resemblance to its film or stage counterparts. Even so, hypnosis is still a fringe activity as far as most Western doctors are concerned. They are not trained to do it, and some of them look on it with undisguised suspicion. One man who doesn't take this view is the Manchester gastroenterologist, Dr Peter Whorwell.

Looking through the medical literature on hypnosis, he discovered accounts, some of them no more than anecdotal, of its use in a variety of conditions including high blood pressure, asthma, and migraine. But no one, it seemed, had reported a careful trial of hypnosis for irritable bowels. Dr Whorwell decided to give it a go.

To make sure he really was putting hypnosis to the test, he chose thirty patients whose symptoms were severe, who had been under his or his colleagues' care for at least a year, and who had failed to respond to any other treatment. Because he was aiming to do a controlled, scientific study of hypnosis, he divided the patients randomly into two groups. One group would receive hypnosis, the other would not. By this means he would be able to assess the true benefits of hypnosis.

Unfortunately, proving that a medical treatment really works is trickier than it might seem. The difficulty stems from the phenomenon I've already mentioned a few times, the placebo effect. The human body has a remarkable and often unexploited capacity to heal itself. One force which galvanizes the body into doing just this is a person's expectation that a particular treatment *will* be beneficial. For example, if a hundred people with headaches are given doses of aspirin, perhaps seventy of them will say that their headaches feel easier within the next hour or so. If you then give another hundred people tablets which they have been told will help their headaches, but which are in fact dummy pills, at least twenty or thirty of this group too will report some lessening of the pain. It wasn't what was in the tablets which did the trick; it was the takers' faith in the tablets which somehow mobilized their bodies' own capacity to overcome the headache.

Such are the problems facing the doctor who is intent on proving that his treatment really works. The particular difficulty when doing a controlled trial of hypnosis is to find a satisfactory placebo for use in the control or comparison group. It's easy enough when you're testing a new drug; you simply give half the patients the dummy pill, but without letting anyone know who has got the real tablets, and who the fake ones. Researchers would like to use this same principle when testing any new therapy. But with something like hypnosis it isn't so easy. To give half of a group of patients a sham form of hypnosis wouldn't work; people may not know what is in a dummy pill, but they know whether or not they have been hypnotized.

To get round this problem, Dr Whorwell had to find a compromise. The patients who weren't chosen to receive hypnosis were instead offered an equal number of half-hour sessions of what he describes as psychotherapy. During these periods, patients discussed their symptoms, and any events in their lives which had proved to be stressful or emotionally upsetting, and might therefore be exacerbating their irritable bowels. They were also given pills to take at regular intervals. Unknown to the patients, these were actually dummies. The point was to create a strong (albeit not identical) placebo effect, and so make sure that the hypnotherapy – if it worked – really was offering something more than the placebo effect alone.

The hypnotherapy patients underwent their treatment in seven half-hour sessions over a period of three months. Before he started the course, Dr Whorwell gave all his patients a brief account of the muscles of the gut, and what they're supposed to do. He next explained the principles of hypnosis, and tried to iron out any misconceptions they might have had. He then demonstrated the technique on someone else; originally he used his secretary, who was not only a good hypnotic subject, but also herself suffered mildly from the syndrome.

How hypnosis is induced

There are many different methods of inducing hypnosis. In one of the commonest, the patient settles himself comfortably before progressively relaxing his body, part by part, as the therapist identifies them: hands, arms, shoulders and so on. With eyes closed, the patient then has to imagine something he finds calming. The better the patient's imagination, the more effective this will be.

A rather impressive variant of this initial phase of inducing hypnosis is called the arm levitation technique. The therapist first tells the patient to place his hand flat on, for example, the arm of the chair, and stare at it. He encourages the patient to concentrate more and more intensely on the hand, and then begins to suggest what might be felt within it. One of these suggestions is that the hand is becoming lighter and lighter. If all goes well, the patient will find his hand beginning to rise, as if by itself. Under the therapist's guidance, he will then be instructed to let his hand drift over to touch his face. As soon as this happens, his arm will fall to his side, his eyes will close, and he will be deeply relaxed.

The next phase of the procedure involves what is known as a 'deepening' process. This might be a minute or so of complete silence; or the therapist may count slowly, while periodically telling the patient how increasingly relaxed he is; or the patient may be told to imagine himself descending in a lift, floor by floor, until it reaches ground level. Variants on this theme are limited only by the imagination of the two parties.

With his patients in a suitably deep trance, Dr Whorwell gave them some fairly general suggestions about how well and healthy they were feeling. He directed their attention to the control of their gut muscles. He asked each patient to place his hand over his abdomen, and to feel a sense of warmth in that area. He then told them to assert control over the activity of their guts; the patients had, as it were, to will their bowels to relax. He asked them to form a mental picture of their intestines if they found this to be helpful.

When judging whether or not the technique worked, Dr Whorwell had one of his colleagues assess the state of each patient's illness. He also had them keep daily diaries in which they rated the frequency and severity of their abdominal pain and distension on a numerical scale of zero to three. They also recorded the normality or otherwise of their bowel habit, the changes in any other symptoms they may have had, and their overall wellbeing.

The benefits of hypnosis

By the end of the three-month period during which the patients kept their scores, the differences between the two groups had become quite dramatic. The control group – the patients who had received psychotherapy – showed an improvement in all symptoms, except their bowel habit. But this improvement was small. By contrast, the symptoms of all fifteen patients who had undergone hypnosis were reduced to score ratings of 'mild'. The difference between the two groups had reached statistical significance (in other words, it could no longer be accounted for by chance alone) within four or five weeks of the start of the treatment: a remarkably rapid rate of progress.

In a further study of hypnotherapy, Dr Whorwell followed up another set of patients for eighteen months. At the end of this time their symptoms were still greatly reduced. Another feature of this study was the importance of the patient's age. Those under fifty responded best – which is fortunate as this group accounts for a disproportionate number of people with the irritable bowel syndrome.

Even Dr Whorwell was taken aback by his findings. As he says, doctors are trained to give medicines and expect results. But it's still rather uncanny when something slightly unconventional gives a good response!

It's tempting to suspect that had Dr Whorwell been using a drug treatment instead of hypnosis, results as clear cut as this (in a group of patients who had failed to respond to all previous medical treatment) would have resulted in a rapid change in clinical practice. In fact it hasn't. In part, of course, this reflects the medical professions's reluctance to get involved with what many of them see as a strictly fringe activity. But that's only part of the problem. As Dr Whorwell himself admits, the major drawback to hypnosis is the time it takes. Even if it was used only for patients who had failed to respond to other treatments, it would still soak up a large amount of practitioner time.

Some saving could be had by teaching patients auto-hypnosis. Using taped instructions, many people find that they can induce a sort of hypnotic trance in themselves without the help of a therapist. But this is most effective as a follow-up technique; it doesn't get round the need for an initial treatment.

In the same issue of the medical journal The Lancet, in which Dr Whorwell reported his findings, an editorial raised one quibble, but otherwise offered some broadly sympathetic support. The quibble concerned the relatively poor improvement achieved by the control group: the patients who had received not hypnosis but psychotherapy. Other people who have tried this technique have sometimes obtained results rather better than those of Dr

Whorwell. So the relatively much greater improvement in Dr Whorwell's hypnotherapy group, though real enough, may not be quite as striking as it appears.

That aside, *The Lancet* went on to say that if patients who had undergone hypnosis really were able to get by without constant and despairing visits to GPs' surgeries and hospital outpatient departments, the investment of time required to make hypnosis work would be amply repaid.

Of course, it could still be argued that the improvement in the patients was less to do with hypnosis as a technique than with some unrealized personal attribute of Dr Whorwell's. He it was who had done all the hypnotizing; maybe it was something about his personality, and not the hypnosis itself, which had helped the patients.

This now seems not to be the case – but it was five years before the medical journals published any other formal study of hypnosis for the irritable bowel syndrome. When one did eventually appear, it came from a group of doctors in Bristol. They used much the same approach as Dr Whorwell, but with one important exception; some of the patients received not individual but group hypnotherapy.

Although the Bristol doctors describe their results as 'less striking' than those obtained by Dr Whorwell, they too found that hypnotherapy was beneficial. Thirty-three of their patients completed the course of treatment, and twenty of them reported an improvement in their symptoms. Indeed, eleven of the twenty were virtually free of symptoms by the end of the study. Because they had used two hypnotherapists, the Bristol doctors were able to compare the results obtained by one with those of the other. There was little difference – implying that what counts is the hypnosis, not just the person doing it.

The Bristol experiment with the use of group hypnosis is particularly important because it suggests that this form of treatment could be made less demanding of expensive professional time. Each group comprised five to seven patients, and relied on the same techniques used in the individual sessions. The only difference was that patients taking part in group sessions discussed their treatment with each other, and exchanged advice. To that extent they had the benefit of mutual support. But the final analysis of the scores showed no differences between the results of group and individual therapy.

Why it works

Why should hypnosis work? The short answer is that no one knows. Two broad explanations seem to offer themselves. One is that hypnosis could be having a non-specific psychological effect. It could be calming the patients, allaying their fears, and generally reassuring them. Dr Whorwell doubts that this is the explanation. In a pilot study he has carried out, hypnosis was at first used only to encourage patients to feel relaxed. Their scores for wellbeing increased – but there was no change in their bowel symptoms until they had received further sessions devoted specifically to the control of gut motility. Dr Whorwell interprets this as meaning that hypnotherapy can have a direct effect on the workings of the gut.

Some attempts to explain why hypnosis works make extravagant use of terms such as the 'consciousness continuum'. They describe how the hypnotist is effectively conducting the patient to deeper levels of consciousness: levels which would otherwise remain, for the most part, inaccessible. The only problem with explanations like this is that they explain nothing. They are simply a conceptual description of what is self-evidently occurring. They tell you nothing of the pattern of electrical activity or of the myriad chemical interactions which take place continually in the nerves of our brains, and must undergo some measurable and possibly profound change during the trance state.

Anyone with a rudimentary knowledge of the organization of the body's nervous system and the way in which individual nerve cells function can devise impressive and sometimes plausible explanations for hypnosis. But in the absence of any hard data, such efforts are largely without value. For the present, we simply to have to accept that hypnosis, like so much else about the brain and nervous system, is a mystery.

However hypnosis works, it has the great virtue of being pretty safe. Disregard the horror stories which appear from time to time about hypnotists taking control of their subjects' minds. The only patients for whom it might represent a threat are those with a psychiatric illness or a history of emotional disturbance. But the careful use of hypnosis to treat a condition like the irritable bowel syndrome seems unlikely to create problems. The aims of the therapist are, after all, quite modest; he's not embarking on some kind of fishing expedition inside the patient's unconscious.

The practicalities of actually getting hypnotherapy aren't always straightforward. The first thing to be said is that it's not wise to make your own diagnosis of this or any other non-trivial illness. You may be convinced, on the basis of the symptoms you've got, that you're suffering from the irritable bowel syndrome. But you may be wrong. So start by seeing your GP and, initially at least, follow whatever advice he gives you. He may decide to treat you himself; or he may refer you to a gastroenterologist at the local hospital. Neither of them is likely to begin treatment by offering you hypnotherapy. Indeed, given the relatively limited number of doctors who know anything about it, it is unlikely that you will be offered hypnotherapy at all.

If the treatment you are receiving doesn't seem to be having any effect, suggest hypnotherapy. Don't be too surprised if your doctor is unenthusiastic. But don't be deterred. Ask him if he can refer you to someone else within the Health Service who is familiar with the technique. Failing that, ask if he knows of anyone practising outside the NHS.

If this gets you nowhere, you're on your own. Hypnotherapists advertise in local papers – but ask for details of his or her training and qualifications (and charges) before you sign up. There is, unfortunately, no legally authorized register of qualified hypnotherapists, so it remains a question of *caveat emptor* – let the buyer beware. There are, however, bodies which keep lists of practitioners, and sometimes set their own standards. The addresses at the back of this book may be helpful. Of course, membership of one of the several professional associations is no more a guarantee of honesty and competence than is membership of, for example, the British Medical Association – but it's better than nothing.

9 Other Psychological Treatments

> To expect us to feel 'humble' in the
> presence of astronomical dimensions
> because they are big is a kind of snobbery
> ... what is significant is mind.
>
> Lord Samuel

In view of the way that our states of mind can affect the workings of our guts, it is hardly surprising that hypnotherapy isn't the only attempt which doctors have made to treat the irritable bowel syndrome using psychological methods. The simplest of these is reassurance. Because this should be part of any therapy for the irritable bowel syndrome – and most other diseases, come to that – it might seem odd to be elevating it to the status of a 'psychological treatment'. It's worth doing so for two reasons: first, to emphasize how important it is; and, second, because the term 'psychological treatment' is really the best description for what reassurance is all about.

An example from elsewhere in medicine best illustrates the remarkable power of reassurance. It concerns an attempt to help patients cope with the pain they would normally experience following an operation, particularly at the place where the surgeon made his incision. One group of patients were prepared for their operation in the usual way. Their surgeons visited them before the operation, but made no special effort to talk about the pain they might expect to feel after they had recovered from the anaesthetic. A similar group of patients were then given detailed information about what to expect, and how to prepare for it. They were told how best to mini- mize the discomfort, and that pain-killing drugs would be available if they were needed. After the operation had been performed, patients who had been reassured in this way requested only half as much medication as those who had received no special preparation; and they were able to leave hospital earlier.

Why should reassurance from the doctor matter so much? Part of the explanation is obvious enough. IBS patients benefit from being assured that their illness is not life-threatening: in particular, that they do not have cancer. But there is more to reassurance than this. There can be hardly a disease in which it's of no value, even when – objectively, at any rate – there is little enough to reassure the patient about. In a terminal illness, when all concerned know there is nothing which can affect the outcome, a reassuring doctor will still be able to offer comfort. But most illnesses – and least of all the irritable bowel syndrome – are not terminal.

Reassurance seems to do more than put the patient's mind at rest, and help him or her cope with the illness (though this, of course, is itself important). It does seem to contribute to the capacity of the patient to recover from the illness. The explanation, surely, is that good doctors act as healers. Just as medical researchers have to discount the placebo effect to evaluate the physical consequences of their treatments, so doctors should be seeking to exploit the effect. The reassurance provided by a good doctor can act as a stimulus to the body's own capacity for self-repair. It is very difficult to define the qualities of the doctor's personality and behaviour which generate this effect. But it is clear that the doctor who doesn't greet his patient, who doesn't look at him during the consultation, who grunts when he should be talking, and who behaves as if he's dealing not with a person but with a disease on legs (does this portrait seem familiar?) is unlikely to generate any health-promoting responses in his patients. The doctor who consciously avoids behaving like this is being more than polite; he is, even though it may not seem like it at the time, psychologically 'treating' his patients.

Several researchers have tried to measure the benefits of using more formal psychological treatments, mostly psychotherapy. This word covers a multitude of different things: some forms of psychotherapy are highly structured, and take their inspiration from one of the schools of psychoanalysis; others are so loose as to resemble nothing more than a rather prolonged chat. What they all have in common is that they rely not on physical intervention, but on verbal encounters between patient and therapist. Hence the collective term sometimes used to describe them: 'talking treatments'.

Talking treatments

The aim of talking treatments is, broadly, to make people more aware of their inner selves: their drives, motives, aspirations and fears. All such treatments – as their name implies – rely on discussion between the patient and a trained therapist. In a series of sessions, each lasting anything from fifteen minutes to an hour, the patients will be asked to talk not only about the problem for which they need help, but about their day-to-day lives, their past experiences, their relationships, their fears, worries and pleasures ... the list is inexhaustible. The therapist will listen, perhaps take notes, and pursue every lead which might have some relevance to (in this case) the roots of the IBS. This may make psychotherapy sound like a forced interrogation – but it isn't. A skilled therapist may actually say very little. Some will encourage you to form your own interpretation of what you reveal; others may lead you to accept theirs. A lot of this form of treatment is administered on a one-to-one basis: just the therapist and you. But psychotherapy can also take the form of a group discussion in which other participants as well as the therapist question, comment, and offer their interpretations. In so far as psychotherapy requires you to confront your true self, it may prove to be something of an ordeal.

In the end, so the argument goes, patients will reach a better understanding of their relationships to the people they know, the environment in which they live, and their feelings about themselves; eventually they should be able to improve these relationships. In so far as these things have a bearing on the cause of their irritable bowel, the improvement should help.

There's no very clear point at which reassurance leaves off and psychotherapy begins; the one may merge insensibly into the other. A great deal of psychotherapy for the irritable bowel syndrome goes on – though not necessarily under that name. You may recall that Dr Whorwell's study of hypnosis (described in the previous chapter) included a comparison group of patients who received what he called psychotherapy. These patients did improve – though not a great deal, and certainly not as much as those who'd received hypnosis. But this study by itself isn't a sufficient basis on which to judge all psychotherapy. For one thing Dr Whorwell's main interest was in hypnosis, not in psychotherapy; it's unlikely he'd thought out this treatment in as much detail as he had the hypnotherapy. And for another, a single study is no basis for judging anything – especially when evaluating a treatment like psychotherapy which comes in so many varieties. In fact, only a few doctors have organized and published studies of its benefits. The two described here should serve to give you an idea of what's involved, and what can come out of it.

One study reported about ten years ago was set up by Dr Ian Hislop working in Fremantle, Western Australia. He set out to record the progress of some sixty patients, most of whom he had given just one or two hours of psychotherapy. The treatment sessions took the form of interviews cum discussions between patient and therapist. Some of the territory covered by Dr Hislop is much the sort of ground which would be turned over in any consultation for the irritable bowel syndrome. He asked patients to give a detailed account of their gut symptoms, and then to describe anything else about their bodily functions or their feelings which was troubling them. He was on the lookout for such things as insomnia, fatigue, loss of libido, anxiety or changes of mood. During this time he tried to establish a good rapport with the patients, and make them feel that he was there to help them.

He went on to find out if anything about their lives was causing them undue stress, or if any particularly upsetting event had happened during the six months before their symptoms began. He asked patients if they had suffered any major loss or deprivation during childhood. While these interviews were in progress, he tried to form an impression of each patient's personality and emotional defences. More positively, he also aimed to get them to express any emotions they might have been repressing. Confronting such emotions is frequently painful, and some patients apparently found themselves reduced to tears. However, Dr Hislop did round things off by making a positive effort to boost their self-esteem.

This is quite an ambitious programme for a course of treatment which might last only a couple of hours. It explains why Dr Hislop took pains to title his treatment 'very brief psychotherapy'. I rather suspect that many specialist psychotherapists would protest against the use of the word psychotherapy, with or without the qualifying 'very brief', to describe so cursory an affair – the more so as Dr Hislop admitted that he'd had no formal training in these skills.

Putting that to one side, Dr Hislop contacted his patients some while after the last session – on average twenty-two months – to find out how they were doing. Each person was asked to fill in a questionnaire designed to find out if the symptoms had improved, and if so by how much. The answers revealed that no patient's symptoms had become worse, and that nearly half the patients had experienced an improvement or were back to normal.

This seems quite impressive. But it has to be remembered that there was no control group by which to judge this progress. How much of this improvement was due to Dr Hislop's efforts, and how much a simple consequence of the disorder curing itself? This study doesn't tell us. All that can be said is that this brief attempt to persuade patients to unburden themselves of anything that was upsetting or worrying them seemed to have had some effect. Dr Hislop was writing as one of those who believe that the irritable bowel syndrome is a bodily manifestation of subconscious emotions generated by recent loss or stressful life events. The results, in his opinion, served to confirm that view. He didn't accept that reassurance alone could have accounted for the improvement.

This, of course, was simply Dr Hislop's conclusion; others would interpret the findings in different ways. But at the very least the study suggests that psychological treatments can sometimes have an effect large enough to make them worthwhile.

Another study of psychotherapy

A more sophisticated exploration of psychotherapy appeared three years later in The Lancet. This study was a collaborative effort between psychiatrists and gastroenterologists from the University of Göteborg in Sweden. These researchers did use a control group; so when they were assessing their results, they were able to compare patients who had undergone psychotherapy with a similar group who had not. Another important difference between this study and its predecessor was that all patients went on receiving conventional medical treatment including bulking agents, drugs, or whatever else was felt to be appropriate. The psychotherapy was not an alternative to medical treatment, but an addition to it.

The psychotherapy itself took the form of a course of ten one-hour sessions over a period of three months, each session conducted by a trained therapist. The treatment was designed to identify emotional problems or sources of stress in each patient's life, find ways of dealing with them, and then set goals which patients might realistically achieve within the period of the course. The treatment didn't end at this point. Thereafter patients were encouraged to go on setting goals, and trying to attain them.

At the end of the three months, and then a year later, the researchers used questionnaires to assess their patients' bodily symptoms – in other words the severity of their IBS – and their state of mind. At three months they found that the psychotherapy patients were experiencing fewer bodily symptoms and were in a better state of mind than those who'd had only medical treatment. A year later, the psychotherapy group's bodily symptoms had improved even more. Patients who had received medical treatment alone showed some deterioration in their condition. Patients in the psychotherapy group also rated themselves as feeling better able to cope with life.

The Swedes who mounted the study conclude that the best way of treating the irritable bowel syndrome is to use a combination of physical and psychological treatment. Given that there does seem to be a psychological element in the IBS, this is eminently sensible. This approach stands in contrast to Dr Hislop's approach in which the irritable bowel syndrome was categorized as a wholly rather than a partly psychosomatic disorder.

Psychotherapy is available through the British NHS, much of it given by clinical psychologists. There are, however, too few of them to meet all demands. Indeed, if gastroenterologists started referring more than a small proportion of their IBS patients for formal treatment by their psychologist colleagues, it seems very probable that the system would be quite unable to cope.

A final point: don't be offended if the doctor suggests that psychotherapy might be appropriate. You shouldn't take that to mean he thinks there's nothing really wrong with you. Nor is there anything to be upset about if at least one of the causes of your particular problem is plainly psychiatric. The notion that psychiatric illness is something to be ashamed of dates from times of witchcraft, superstition, and ignorance about the nature and workings of the human body. If you meet people who think otherwise, scorn their attitudes as outmoded, and their opinions as worthless!

Stress management

The importance of stress in provoking attacks of the irritable bowel syndrome is open to dispute; but assuming that it could play a role of some kind, it's worth considering ways of trying to overcome it. There are several approaches which have been devised in an effort to help deal with stress; a couple of examples will serve to give the flavour of these methods. One of the simplest is progressive muscle relaxation. The subject repeatedly, methodically, and quite slowly tenses and relaxes each major group of muscles, while concentrating on the sensation within them. During a session lasting perhaps twenty-five minutes, each group of muscles might be tensed and relaxed two or three times. It is possible to buy taped instructions to be played while doing the exercise. To make the most of progressive muscle relaxation the patient has to learn to recognize the onset of feelings of tension, and use the muscle relaxation technique before those feelings get the better of him. In the longer term, of course, it is necessary to identify those situations which tend to induce stress, and then change things accordingly. The hard evidence that these methods are effective is extremely limited; they tend to be more popular with psychologists and psychiatrists than with gastroenterologists. But some patients do find them helpful, and I'll have more to say on stress and what you can do about it in the next chapter.

Biofeedback

Biofeedback can be used simply as another, rather more technological method of stress management. In principle, all biofeedback techniques depend on subjects being given information about their bodies which isn't normally available to them. A simple example can be found in the treatment of high blood pressure by this method. The level of our blood pressure isn't normally under our conscious control – though we do know that being calm and relaxed tends to lower it. The biofeedback technique allows the user to exert more direct, more methodical control. The trick is to let subjects know, moment by moment, how relaxed they are. This can be done by connecting electrodes to, for example, the small muscles in the forehead. As the whole body becomes relaxed, so too do these particular muscles. This can be detected by the electrodes. The electrical signals these record are then revealed to the subject in one of several ways. It could be visual (a needle moving across a meter to indicate the tension of the muscles) or auditory (a soft continuous note that rises or falls according to the subjects' state of relaxation). With this information being relayed to them, most people soon find that they can consciously and fairly predictably induce a state of relaxation, and thereafter a fall in their blood pressure.

The evidence that biofeedback relaxation also minimizes the symptoms of the IBS is not exactly overwhelming; but some sufferers have apparently found it helpful. Not satisfied with this non-specific role for biofeedback, a couple of attempts have been made to make more specific use of it. One researcher has used signals recorded from the subjects' own intestines. Each patient in this particular experiment had to agree to the insertion of a balloon through the anus, and up into the large bowel. A tube attached to the balloon was then used to inflate it, so exerting outward pressure on the wall of the bowel and inducing it to contract, just as it would if full of faeces. Contractions of the gut were recorded by electrodes and relayed to the subjects. Thus each had a continuous indication of the activity of his own gut. Two thirds of a group of patients were able to learn to control their gut motility in a single two-hour session. Eight weeks later they were still able to demonstrate this remarkable talent. Whether they were able to make good use of it in overcoming their IBS symptoms isn't clear.

Still more intriguingly – and rather less messily –

another researcher used an electronic stethoscope to allow sufferers to listen to an amplified version of their own bowel sounds. The doctor who pioneered this remarkable enterprise claimed that his patients could not only learn to influence their bowel activity, but that it helped reduce their symptoms. Others who've tried to replicate the work have been less impressed. Still, it does demonstrate the value of ingenuity when trying to overcome the irritable bowel syndrome.

10 Two Brains in Conflict?

> What good are brains to a man? They
> only unsettle him.
>
> P.G. Wodehouse

Chapter 4 described the role which stress might play in provoking attacks of the irritable bowel syndrome. Elsewhere in this book you will have come across suggestions that the cause of the IBS lies in some abnormality of the workings of the gut itself. One man has tried to put these two views together – and in so doing has come up with yet another way of looking at the irritable bowel syndrome. Professor David Wingate is director of the Gastrointestinal Science Research Unit at the London Hospital. His recent experimental work has followed two main themes: finding out what stress does to the gut; and exploring the link between the central and the enteric nervous systems – or, to put it more slickly, between the big brain in the head, and the little brain in the gut.

In the past couple of decades, stress has become one of the most overworked words in the English language. This is largely because we all use it to mean different things. Anything we find unpleasant, but for which there is no immediately available remedy, we are apt to label 'stressful'. The faintly clinical connotations of the word give an added importance to what might sound rather trivial if described merely as 'worrying' or 'upsetting'. It's a catch-all concept – and as such extremely useful. If the radio starts to play music we don't like, we retune to another station, or turn it off; if the noisy neighbours insist on playing Radio 1 at full blast when the music we like is on Radio 3, this is stress. So is travelling on the London Underground during the rush hour, using a word processor in an un-soundproofed office beside a main road, getting up in the middle of the night to feed the baby, working on a factory production line, going through a marriage break-up, moving house, preparing for an examination, looking after an elderly and demented relative . . . and so on and so on. When a word can be taken to mean so much, it may also be judged to mean very little.

Why should we hear so much of stress nowadays? Think for a moment of the threats and hazards facing one of our long-deceased ancestors: a cave dweller, for example. Imagine that he wakes up in the morning feeling hungry. The task to be accomplished is not a matter of starting the car, driving to the supermarket, and deciding which of several thousand items to buy; rather it's about making and sharpening a spear with which to hunt and kill a possibly dangerous animal – or starve. And when evening comes, and tiredness, there's no climbing the stairs and snuggling under a duvet; there's just a heap of wet bracken to lie on – and before that a fire to be lit in the hope of discouraging animal predators which are every bit as hungry as you. Now that really is what I call stress. Odd, then, that the people who seem perpetually dissatisfied with life, and who seem to suffer the most grumbling, discontented and stressful existences are not Nepali peasants, or Kung Bushmen, or South American

Indians (at least so long as they're living in their traditional manner) but urban people with all the gewgaws and comforts and protections of technological civilization. Why so?

One can only guess – but it probably has something to do with the kind of stresses to which we're subject. Evolution, of course, generously prepared us to face difficult circumstances. As soon as we realize that the fire we lit to deter animal intruders has gone out, and that a wolf is even now snuffling around the fringes of the camp, messages from our brain bring about a series of changes in our body chemistry and physiology which prepare us to do one of two things: fight off the wolf; or, if it looks exceptionally intimidating, shin with all speed up the nearest tree. A few of the hazards of urban living are much as they ever were: so when stopped by a couple of youths asking you to hand over your wallet, the 'fight or flight' response would prove as useful as ever. But look back at those stresses I listed in the last but one paragraph. Many of them – and many more that could have been included – are not open to immediate remedy. If we want to get to work, we may have no option but to travel on the Underground during the rush hours; if we want to work at all, there may be no alternative to the factory production line – and so on.

Each of these experiences, and a great many others, will anger or distress or frighten us; and each will produce some degree of arousal. But if there is nothing then and there to be done, and this physiological arousal can achieve nothing, it serves only to exacerbate our discomfort. What were once a set of useful bodily responses have become mentally and physically irrelevant or, worse, self-damaging. To be confident about which bodily diseases are a product of stress, at least in part, is impossible. Most of the evidence comes from work on heart disease, and on ulcers of the stomach and gut. Even here a lot of the evidence is open to challenge. Stress is as hard to detect and measure as it is to define. Moreover there is the individual's perception of stress to be taken into account. A study on stress and ulcers brought this into sharp relief a few years ago when one of the participants denied that the death of a parent had been stressful. The death of a close relative is one of those experiences generally, and quite reasonably, thought of as creating stress; puzzled, the researchers asked their subject to explain. It emerged that the father had been suffering from a chronic, painful and incurable disease – and the moment of death was a relief for the son as well as the father. A system of determining the existence of stress and rating its severity which takes no account of individual circumstances is likely to give entirely misleading impressions. One person's stress is another's stimulus. This is one reason, no doubt, why a lot of work on stress has proved so contradictory.

To make matters more complicated, there is a theory developed by two Americans, Mayer Friedman and Ray Rosenman, which sees people as having one or other of two personality types called A and B. The type B people are less likely, so it is claimed, to suffer from stress problems. They don't constantly feel the urge to compete; they are relaxed, tolerant and patient. Type A people, on the other hand, are always competing, aggressive, easily roused and thoroughly impatient. Whether anyone has ever analysed irritable bowel patients in terms of this twofold personality type I don't know. It might make an interesting experiment.

Peering into the gut

Back in the late forties, one group of researchers decided to take a direct look directly at what happens in the gut while people are undergoing stress. The first subjects were healthy medical students who agreed to be examined by sigmoidoscopy while enduring various forms of stress including a headband which could be screwed tighter, and continuous immersion of one hand in ice cold water. (It's a serious business, getting a medical degree.) Through the sigmoidoscope the researchers were able to see that these painful stimuli increased the flow of blood through the lining of the colon, and caused its muscles to tighten. These experiments were repeated on IBS patients – whose guts responded more vigorously than did those of otherwise healthy subjects.

The students were also subjected to the mental stress of what is described as an 'unsympathetic interview'. (What an extraordinary sight this experiment would have presented to anyone who blundered uninvited into the laboratory: a man being questioned by an interrogator who directed his questions to one end of the body while apparently seeking his answers at the other!) One hapless student was falsely led to believe that his internal examiner had discovered a tumour – an exceedingly cruel experiment which would nowadays, one hopes, be disallowed by the research ethics committee who would have vetted the planned work. This work revealed that when IBS patients felt hostile, angry or anxious, their gut muscles tightened up and the flow of blood through them increased. Feelings of hopelessness or inadequacy tended to have the opposite effect. It is very difficult to know what to make of these findings, other than the obvious conclusion: that in most people stress can affect bowel function, and that in people with the IBS these responses seem to be exaggerated. Not terribly helpful.

The small intestine

Professor Wingate and colleagues set out to examine the effect of stress on the activity not of the large, but of the small bowel. As they point out, it's difficult to define a pattern even of normal activity in the large bowel; so deciding what constitutes an abnormality is even harder. In the small intestine, by contrast, there are characteristic patterns of contractile activity both at rest, following meals, and in certain types of illness. Professor Wingate measures the activity of the bowel by having his subjects swallow small 'radiotelemetric' capsules. Radiotelemetry is simply a fancy term to describe any process in which data are relayed by radio to the experimenter from a measuring device placed in an otherwise inaccessible location. The capsules used by Professor Wingate contained a device which responded to pressure changes in their surroundings; the more active the muscles of the gut, the greater the variation of the pressure within it. Also inside each capsule was a transmitter able to send this information on pressure changes over a short distance. The distances were, in fact, very short because subjects who had swallowed the capsules had aerials fixed to the skin over their abdomens. Signals from the aerial were fed into a recording device small enough to be strapped around the waist. The tape from this recorder could later be played back through another instrument which displayed the actual changes of pressure within the gut. The virtue of this system was that it allowed the subjects to move about normally more or less unhampered, and not be confined to the laboratory.

To ensure that the capsules went as far down the gut as required, and no further, each was tethered on a length of thread attached at its upper end to the subject's cheek. (The capsules weren't cheap; tethering them also ensured that the research team knew where they were, and could haul them back at the end of the experiment!) Each subject swallowed two capsules, the pair being separated along the thread by a distance of 15 centimetres (6 inches). Because the capsules were swallowed after an overnight fast, they moved quite rapidly through the stomach and into the duodenum. Using fluoroscopy (a kind of X-ray viewing system) the researchers were able to tell when the capsules had reached their appointed location in the upper reaches of the small bowel.

Professor Wingate's study of each subject lasted for just over thirty hours. He started recording their gut motility on the morning of the first day. During this time participants were free to read or to watch television; they were not, however, free to eat. No food was allowed until the evening; at that time they were given a standard meal containing a set number of calories. On day two of the experiment they again had to fast. They also had to undergo three periods of stress: two in the morning and one in the afternoon. The stress came in three forms, each lasting two hours. The first involved driving a car through the streets of London: stress indeed. A second required subjects to play an electronic video game called Asteroids. The object is to pilot a spaceship out of the path of asteroids and other, hostile craft. As this is intended by the manufacturers to be a game, and not a source of stress, the choice may seem puzzling. But most games requiring intense concentration pall when played for two hours to the accompaniment of noisy sound effects. The third task utilized a technique called 'delayed audio feedback'. The subject, wearing headphones, reads aloud into a microphone. The wiring is such that the sound of his voice is fed back into his own headphones. This innocent set-up is rendered treacherous by introducing a quarter-second delay into the signal entering the headphones. Anyone who has tried to speak while hearing his own voice coming back to him with a slight delay will know something of the determined concentration required to keep going. The effect is like that of having a physical brake applied to the speaking voice: most disconcerting.

The subjects themselves fell into three groups: IBS patients; normal healthy adults; and patients with organic bowel disease. The reason for having this last group was to ensure that any abnormalities found in the IBS patients couldn't be dismissed as a response common to all diseases of the gut, and having no connection with the irritable bowel syndrome in particular. Once the data on gut motility had been printed out, Professor Wingate was able to compare the frequency of the migrating motor complexes (the fancy name for the regular bursts of muscular activity in the small bowel) in the various patient groups before and during stress. In nineteen out of the twenty-two IBS patients in the study he found one or more abnormalities; of the normal healthy subjects only one was abnormal; of the patients with organic bowel disease, all were normal as far as gut activity was concerned.

More specifically, all three groups showed the same frequency of bowel contractions during the first twenty-four hours of the study. When the stress sessions began, they affected all subjects – but not in the same way. In the normal subjects, and in the patients with organic disease, stress induced the gut muscles to contract twice as often. By contrast, in many of the IBS patients gut activity virtually stopped altogether, or gave way to prolonged and abnormal contractions. During the fast period, a large proportion of the IBS patients also experienced phases of irregular contraction lasting from one to six hours. In women, stress more often evoked this irregular activity.

The measurement methods used by Professor Wingate are so unobtrusive that he has since studied a number of patients in their own homes. When patients come into hospital their symptoms sometimes disappear, perhaps because they are removed from the domestic or occupational stresses which Professor Wingate thinks provoke them. Hence the need for artificial stresses like the video game to bring them on again. When the experiments were repeated on patients going about their normal daily lives, the irregular periods of contractions appeared again, and were often associated with symptoms of which the patients themselves were aware. Interestingly the irregular contractions were confined to the waking period; generally they stopped as soon as the patients fell asleep.

Big and little

How, then, to account for these findings? Professor Wingate frames his explanation in terms of the relationship between the enteric and the central nervous systems. Chapter 1 described how the brain exerts its influence over the gut by (among other means) a group of nerves known collectively as the parasympathetic system. One of these, the vagus nerve, has traditionally been thought of as having a particularly important influence on the gut. That view has been overturned by research showing that the vast majority of the bundle of individual nerve fibres which make up the vagus nerve carry information not from the brain to the gut, but in the other direction: from the gut to the brain. In any one nerve fibre, messages run only in one direction. In short, the brain has many more channels of communication for finding out what is happening in the gut than it has for influencing these events. With so few channels available there is no way that the brain could take immediate charge of the immensely intricate sequence of co-ordinated contractions required to ensure that the gut functions as it should. This is what makes Professor Wingate believe that most of what goes on in the gut is the result of activity locally initiated and locally co-ordinated – by the enteric nervous system. When the big brain seeks to influence gut activity, it does so by delivering a message to the little brain: to the enteric nervous system. It might, for example, instruct the gut to switch from one pre-programmed type of activity to another – typically from 'between meals' behaviour to 'food arriving' behaviour.

Both brains are necessary for normal and appropriate

gut function. Cut the gut's links to the central nervous system and its actions will no longer be tuned to the needs of the body it is supposed to serve. Conversely, destroy the enteric nervous system and the result is a loss of organized function and a descent into random and disorganized bursts of contraction. There are indeed one or two known organic diseases in which precisely this seems to be the cause of the problem. An example is – sorry about this – 'chronic idiopathic intestinal pseudo-obstruction'. This needs taking apart: 'chronic' means that it goes on a long time; 'idiopathic' is a medical euphemism for 'cause unknown'; 'intestinal pseudo-obstruction' means that while the patient's symptoms seem to suggest that something must be blocking the gut, there is no physical obstruction to be found. Some cases of this disorder appear to result from an abnormality of the gut muscles; but in other cases the fault seems to lie in a degeneration of the enteric nerves. This is good evidence of the importance of the enteric nervous system in keeping gut motility operating smoothly.

Enter stress

Professor Wingate describes the relationship between the big brain and little brain as a kind of dialogue in which the latter is subservient to the former. When the brain perceives that its circumstances are stressful, it sends messages which alter gut function. We must assume that the changes so brought into play were, to our ancestors, of some survival value. Putting all this together, Professor Wingate suggests that what is happening in IBS patients is that the big brain is interfering with the actions of the little brain. The form that this interference might take is a matter of speculation. There are a number of options to choose from. A brain experiencing stress could start delivering too many messages, or sending confused or incorrect ones. Or the fault could lie in the enteric nervous system; the messages which all our brains send out during stress might be perfectly standard, but for some reason the enteric nervous systems of IBS patients respond too vigorously, or otherwise incorrectly. All sorts of parallels come to mind if you think of the big brain as a telephone exchange, and the little brain as the handset in your own home. If your phone doesn't ring when someone is trying to reach you, you can't tell whether the fault lies within your handset or at the exchange. In the former case the correct signal is reaching your home, but not being acted upon; in the latter case, where the fault lies centrally, the signal itself is scrambled or missing altogether. But, as I say, it's all speculation.

Such thoughts are of more than merely academic interest because they point the way to new methods of diagnosing and treating the irritable bowel. Measurement techniques of the kind used by Professor Wingate would make it possible for the first time to develop an objective method of recognizing the IBS. No longer would clinicians have to rely on a system of diagnosis which depends on nothing more positive than eliminating everything else. Even assuming that the IBS isn't all of a piece, it would then be possible to distinguish between patients in whom there was some abnormality of the nerve supply to the gut, and others in whom the problem was primarily, say, psychological. As far as treatment is concerned, the drugs currently available have proved to be less than impressive. If Professor Wingate is correct, there might be something to be gained by developing a drug which would reduce or eliminate the interference of the big brain with the programmes of gut contraction being run by the little brain. This might be a drug which acted centrally – in the brain, that is – or locally, in the gut. All of which is easy enough to propose, but difficult to put into practice. It is likely that a good deal more will have to be learned about this link between the brain and gut before some kind of intervention can be devised. And all this, of course, depends on Professor Wingate's ideas turning out to be correct.

One specialist in the nervous control of the gut has compared the state of development of his branch of medicine to that reached by neurology around the turn of the century. At that time disorders like Parkinson's disease could only be categorized as 'functional'. The patient's symptoms – the muscular tremor, the rigidity, and the rest of them – were only too evident; but the doctors had no way of knowing what might be causing them. Eventually it was possible to demonstrate chemical and physical abnormalities in the brains of people suffering from Parkinsonism. Now there are treatments. Admittedly these are far from perfect, and in no way to be described as cures. But Parkinson's disease is no longer numbered among the functional diseases because we have begun to pin down its cause. In this instance it was the careful unravelling of the chemistry of the big brain which paid dividends; gastroenterologists – or those at least who believe that nervous system failures lie at the root of the IBS – are confident that something similar will happen to bring relief to irritable bowel syndrome patients.

11 Alternative Medicine and the IBS

> George Prendergast was sitting cross-legged on the floor in the middle of his office, with his hands on his knees.
>
> 'What are you doing?' Vic demanded.
>
> 'Breathing', said Prendergast, getting to his feet. 'Yoga breathing exercises for my irritable bowel syndrome.'
>
> 'You look daft, if you don't mind my saying so.'
>
> 'It helps, though,' said Prendergast.
>
> David Lodge, *Nice Work*

In the beginning there was fringe medicine. But although the term was devised by a sympathizer, its advocates came to dislike what they saw as the offensive connotations of the word 'fringe'. So 'fringe medicine' became 'alternative medicine', the implication being that here was a collection of treatments distinctly different from those on offer from orthodox medicine. But this still wasn't quite right – not least because it fostered the accusation that alternative practitioners saw themselves as being in competition with orthodox medicine, and might therefore be tempted to 'steal' patients whose maladies would be more appropriately dealt with by the GP or the surgeon. Hence the third generation name, complementary medicine. This avoids any suggestion that the patient has to make a choice: either I'm treated by orthodox medicine, or I go to the naturopath, the osteopath, the acupuncturist or whoever it may be. The logic here is that unorthodox practices are intended not to replace conventional treatments, but to use ways of thinking about and dealing with sickness which do not usually form part of conventional practice. It's certainly the case that much of what takes place in the alternative practitioner's consulting room is quite unlike most of what goes on in, for example, the high-tech district general hospital. But because the term 'complementary' has never really caught on to the point at which it can be said to have replaced 'alternative', this book will continue to refer to 'alternative medicine'.

In an ideal world the distinction between 'orthodox' and 'alternative' would be irrelevant. Since the *raison d'être* for all forms of treatment must be that they benefit patients, there should be no requirement to make such a distinction. The need has arisen because there are different and sometimes irreconcilable views about which treatments are beneficial. The diversity of both conventional and alternative medicine is such that it's not easy to summarize in a few words what both camps think they are about. However, conventional medicine today is in essence scientific medicine. And alternative medicine has flourished as a kind of rebellion against a widespread public perception of scientific medicine as lacking in humanity.

The introduction of scientific thought to medicine was not immediately popular. For centuries physicians had relied largely on the writings of ancient authorities such as Hippocrates and Galen. Their works were not looked on in the way that we might view such treatises: as provisional statements of knowledge, valid at the time they were written. Rather they were regarded more as the medical equivalent of a holy book like the Bible or the Koran: a definitive statement of the way things are. The words might be open to reinterpretation, but few people – least of all physicians – felt it appropriate to challenge them, root and branch. Then, as now, physicians made a good living: they did, after all, have a handful of genuinely useful remedies; while many of the potions they dispensed did no particular good, neither did most of them do a great deal of harm; they had the placebo effect on their side; and the physicians' patients, of course, were even more ignorant and credulous than were they themselves. Why should the doctors wish to upset what was, for them, a moderately successful apple cart?

In the end, of course, the obvious achievements of science made it virtually inevitable that this way of looking at the world would invade medicine as much as it has most other human enterprises. The essential feature of science is its method of acquiring and evaluating knowledge. Revelation, divine or otherwise, is out; its replacement is careful observation and painstaking experiment. Facts are no longer treated as such simply because a Galen or a Hippocrates declared them to be so. Science demands verification. A claim is only as sound as the strength of the last attempt made to test it. All knowledge is provisional: a statement of things as we understand them today, and an acknowledgement that tomorrow or the day after, in the light of new evidence, we may have to change our minds. In practice, of course, science is practised not by machines, but by men; so that perfect model is seldom followed to the letter. Science is no less prey to competition and petty jealousies than are other human affairs. What makes science unique as a way of looking at the world is its inbuilt necessity to criticize its own understandings, to abandon ideas which have been tested and failed, and to find more robust ideas and explanations. These changes, as they happen, may threaten and cause pain to individuals; but science itself is strengthened.

Negative views of science

This is not, alas, how everyone sees science. There are, of course, whole areas of human experience to which science has no obvious relevance. It may one day be possible to explain why York Minster or a Beethoven symphony evoke such profound feelings in so many people. For the present it is not possible. As there is no practical necessity to explain these things, they are not areas of great scientific endeavour. Moreover, even among the small number of scientists who do have an academic, professional interest in such questions, fewer still would sit through the choral movement of Beethoven's Ninth wondering how the nerve cells of their brains are transforming the sound patterns of the 'Ode to Joy' into emotional responses. Like the rest of us they are content to embrace the emotion itself without worrying at that particular moment why they feel what they are feeling. For all this, though, science is still seen as antithetical to human values and experiences: as a force which undermines or even devalues them. Science and scientists are still admired – but felt to be slightly lacking in soul, and best kept at arm's length.

As with science, so – to a lesser, though perceptibly increasing extent – with medicine. Despite the evident achievements of medicine, from antibiotics to insulin, the past few decades have seen more and more people beginning to feel less and less comfortable with conventional doctoring. The more that medicine can do in a technical sense (and the more that is expected of it) the more do many people feel that doctors no longer see them as people with problems, but simply as cases. Correctly or not, many patients feel they're treated by the doctor with no more concern for their individuality than might be expected of a car mechanic dealing with an engine. To some degree this is perhaps inevitable. When the state of understanding of the human body was such that the doctor had little he could do in a technical sense, the greater part of the consultation was spent concentrating on the patient as a person. The increasing number of things that doctors could actually do to and for patients meant that an increasing proportion of the consultation time had to be given over to doing these things. Understandably, it is in hospital medicine that such technical innovation has produced the greatest change. Indeed, in some branches of hospital medicine the doctor's role really has become that of 'body mechanic'. This is not the kind of relationship which satisfies patients. If any one thing can be said to epitomize the image of the modern hospital, it's the intensive care unit with its bright lights and its continually humming and bleeping instruments. Even the nurses in such places seem to spend more time watching dials and keeping an eye open for flashing lights than they do talking to and reassuring the bedridden inmates. In such circumstances patients are not only surrounded by machinery, but may feel reduced to the same level of significance: one living machine surrounded by a lot of inanimate ones.

This sense that human values have begun to take a back seat alienates many people who would otherwise have no quibbles with scientific medicine. This might just be bearable if modern medicine was able to fulfil its implied promise of a cure for every ill. Clearly it cannot. The result is a substantial minority of patients who find themselves receiving the worst of both worlds: their physical illness remains uncured, while at the same time they feel they are being denied much of the tender loving care we all need when we are sick. When the seeds of alternative medicine fall on such ground, they find it fertile.

Whole persons

One of the few things that nearly all alternative medical techniques have in common is they they claim to treat specific complaints within the context of the patient as a whole person: the holistic approach, to use the fashionable term. The alternative practitioner will wish to know not just about the disorder which has brought the patient to his consulting room, but also about the workings of the rest of that person's body, and indeed of the rest of his life. In truth this may or may not be relevant; but it is certainly very comforting to anyone accustomed to the usual five minutes with a GP. Of course, the patient visiting an alternative practitioner has every right to expect more than five minutes. He is, after all, most likely paying for it; the health service offers very little in the way of unorthodox therapy.

The claim that orthodox medicine fails to treat disease in its whole-body context has some merit to it – though not as much as most alternative practitioners would have us believe. Some doctors don't look beyond the symptoms of which the patient complains; they don't ask themselves whether wider or deeper problems might be causing the disorder which the patient is telling them about. Good doctors do consider these things as a matter of course – and to that extent are themselves practising holistic medicine. But the average GP or hospital doctor is not going to spend valuable time probing things which he simply doesn't believe to be relevant to the patient's illness.

Another characteristic of alternative medicine – arguably its most admirable – is the encouragement it gives to people to take an active part in improving their own health. In parallel with the rise of scientific medicine there has been an increasing tendency for us to hand all responsibility for our health to the doctor. We visit him when we are sick; he does certain things to or for us, and issues instructions which we (in theory) obey. Our role is essentially passive: the recipient of 'doctor's orders', as the saying has it. A lot of alternative medicine is more demanding; it requires patients to take an active part in their treatments – not so much during consultations as between them. This may involve diet, meditation, relaxation, exercises or any one of a variety of other things.

Ideally, as I have already argued, there should be no need to make distinctions between 'orthodox' and 'alternative' procedures. The only distinction which matters is between procedures which have been shown to work, and procedures which haven't. By this assessment alternative medicine does pretty badly. Most of the evidence called to support it is anecdotal, or otherwise unreliable. Controlled trials of the kind which are routine in orthodox medicine are rare indeed outside it. Some alternative practitioners positively oppose the collection of such evidence, arguing that the required experiments are unnecessary, or even unethical because they 'know' the technique works. Their position is something like that of the man who 'knows' that cigarettes don't cause lung cancer because his granny smoked eighty a day, and lived to be a hundred. It's easy for enthusiastic practitioners (never mind charlatans, of which there are more than a few) to pull out a handful of case histories which 'prove' that the therapies work. If you are shown such evidence, ask about the patients who didn't benefit from the treatment. And remember that there is such a thing as spontaneous recovery. Such are the body's own healing powers that most of the illnesses we contract will clear up of their own accord; why allow an unscrupulous or misguided practitioner to claim the credit for what your own body has managed to do all by itself?

Placebos again

And then, of course, there's our old friend the placebo effect. Any patient who sincerely believes in his practitioner and what is being done for him may benefit by a treatment – even if, in reality, the 'treatment' is no more than a teaspoonful of coloured water. The extent of the benefit will depend on the condition being treated, but it is reckoned that as much as 30 per cent of the improvement achieved by many drugs is a direct consequence of the placebo effect. The greater the part played by the mind in causing or influencing a disease, the potentially greater will be the placebo effect.

Consider the bearing which this can have on, for example, the testing of a new drug for treating the irritable bowel syndrome. In the usual kind of controlled trial, half the patients will be given the active drug, and half a dummy – neither doctor nor patient knowing until the experiment is over who got what. If it turns out the patients who got the active drug have experienced, on average, a 40 per cent reduction in their symptoms the researcher may well feel pleased. This seems to be a drug which can bring about a worthwhile improvement. His pleasure, though, will be short lived if he discovers that the dummy pill alone was able to bring about a 30 per cent improvement: in other words, that most of the improvement was attributable to the placebo effect. Bearing this in mind will help to put what are superficially impressive claims into a more realistic perspective.

One final point: none of this is intended to suggest that alternative treatments aren't worth trying. The fact that something hasn't been proved to work is not the same as saying that it doesn't work. Some alternative techniques may be effective; but it would be quite wrong to recommend them on the grounds that they *have* been demonstrated as effective when in fact they haven't. As a general rule, though, it's sensible to give orthodox medicine a good try before abandoning it – if for no better reason than that through the British NHS (and other medical programmes) you can get most of it without further payment! If conventional medicine fails, then alternative medicine may be a sensible next step. And if this does bring about an improvement, whether it was the procedure itself or its placebo effect which should take the credit is largely academic.

Incidentally, nothing I have said should be taken to mean that everything in orthodox medicine is of proven effectiveness. This is far from the case – treatments for the irritable bowel syndrome being no exception. Not all the remedies offered by the GP and the gastroenterologist will have been subjected to as close a scrutiny as, ideally, they should. A pinch of scepticism is useful in most circumstances. The difference between orthodox and alternative medicine is that orthodox treatments are more *likely* to have been objectively tested, not that they definitely *will* have been.

Three techniques – relaxation, hypnosis and biofeedback – which are often categorized as 'alternative' have already been described in the context of the 'orthodox' treatment sections of this book. This illustrates both the way in which mainstream and alternative medicine overlap, and the essentially artificial nature of the distinction. How many branches of alternative medicine you choose to recognize is a matter of taste. There are maybe a score of broad approaches, each of which has several or many sub-groupings. Alternative medicine, like religion, has a tendency to undergo periodic division. And new methods of treatment keep on turning up. The handful considered in slightly more detail here are somewhat arbitrarily chosen, but do give an indication of the breadth of alternative medicine. They are also among the better known and well-established of what is available. Few honest practitioners would claim that their particular treatment is uniquely suited to the treatment of the irritable bowel syndrome. Most, in fact, would say that their therapies can be of some benefit in conditions of almost every sort. The more reasonable among them will not claim to be able to cure everything; but they will say that even when their systems of medicine cannot compete with conventional methods – in dealing with a broken leg, for example – their treatments will still form a useful adjunct and accelerate the body's own healing processes.

Acupuncture

For many people, I suspect, acupuncture is typical of what alternative medicine is about: it involves doing something (sticking needles in the body) which is decidedly odd; it is very ancient; and it comes from the Orient. All these things render it mysterious and exotic – though in truth acupuncture is becoming so much more commonplace that the wonder is beginning to wear off. There are even some orthodox doctors who offer it. The essence of the procedure is nowadays familiar to most people. The practitioner inserts a number of fine, sterilized needles into specific points on the patient's body selected according to the nature of the disorder which is being treated. In most cases the needles penetrate only to a depth of a few millimetres. The points at which the needles have to be inserted are not necessarily anywhere near the site of the problem under treatment. The needles may be left in place for only a few seconds, or for up to an hour depending on the nature of the treatment. Once the patient has become accustomed to the needles, and is happy with the procedure, the acupuncturist may twirl the needles periodically by rotating them between thumb and forefinger. Most people who haven't had acupuncture imagine it must be painful; indeed, the sight of a cluster of needles sticking out of someone's arm or back can give the observer a sympathy twinge. But a dextrous therapist can insert the needles without causing pain.

There are one or two variants of acupuncture. In

moxibustion, a small cone of a type of dried herb is placed on the skin at the acupuncture point, ignited, and allowed to smoulder. This is allowed to burn down until the patient can feel the heat – but not so far down that it burns the skin. Alternatively the herb cone may be placed on the end of the needle and ignited – the heat then travelling down the needle and into the patient. In a more recent variant of the basic technique, electroacupuncture, a small current is passed through the needles.

According to the traditional theory of acupuncture, the superficial layers of the body incorporate a series of lines or meridians – each of which acts as a channel through which energy is shunted around the body from one place to another. Each meridian serves a particular part or organ of the body. To take a relevant example, the meridian for the colon runs from the tip of the index finger up the arm to the shoulder, then to the neck and the nose and, after plunging into the deeper layers of the body, reaches the colon itself. For acupuncture to be effective, the needles have to be inserted at points along the relevant lines. The position chosen will depend on whether the aim is to disperse or to gather the energy in these lines – and this in turn will be determined by the nature of the patient's illness.

Science finds this explanation unsatisfactory, partly because no one has been able to find any anatomical or physiological evidence of the existence of these lines, and partly because the acupuncturists' concept of energy balance has no meaning in biology and medicine. The manifest effectiveness of acupuncture in certain areas including pain control and anaesthesia has prompted many attempts to find a scientific explanation. One theory is that the needles stimulate the body to release chemicals called 'endorphins'. These are natural counterparts of the opiate drugs such as morphine and heroin, and are thought to have a variety of effects on the body, including the extent to which we perceive pain. But this is just a theory; the evidence is by no means conclusive.

Most acupuncture practitioners are not medically qualified, although in Britain there are about 150 doctors who have studied acupuncture.

Homeopathy

In Britain homeopathy is the most firmly established of the alternative therapies – and the only one with firm NHS recognition. This is sometimes thought to stem from the favour with which the Royal Family is believed to look on homeopathy; in fact its right to exist within the health service was enshrined at the time of its creation. There are now four hundred or so medically qualified homeopaths: individuals whose standing tends to be rather higher with the public than with some at least of their own colleagues.

Many of the fundamental concepts owe their origin to Dr Samuel Hahnemann who published his founding treatise on homeopathy in the early part of the nineteenth century. Underlying it is the principle that 'like cures like'. If a particular illness is characterized by, say, fever, the homeopathic remedies which are most likely to benefit the patient are those which, in a healthy individual, would provoke such symptoms. In an age which has long since accustomed itself to immunization – in which protection against an infectious disease is sought by inoculating the body with all or part of the organism responsible for causing that disease – the notion of like curing like should not seem entirely alien. In reality the parallels between immunization and homeopathy are slender – and dwindle further when you recall the second underlying principle of homeopathy: repeated dilution of the original ingredient. Common sense would suggest that this will make the medicine progressively less effective. But homeopaths claim that the reverse is true: that with dilution it becomes more effective or 'potent', to use the jargon term. These dilutions are not a matter of reducing the concentration of the active ingredient ten or even a hundred fold. The dilution process may be repeated so many times that there are good theoretical reasons to suppose (this is one of the few things which homeopaths and their critics agree on) that not a single molecule of the original ingredient is left in the diluted fluid. Indeed, by standard chemical tests, many homeopathic remedies would show up as pure water – or whatever other fluid has been used to do the dilution.

Another distinguishing feature of the homeopathic remedy is the way in which the dilution is carried out. Each step in the process is accompanied by a vigorous shaking known as 'succussion'. The nearest that homeopaths can come to an explanation of why their remedies work is that the shaking causes the active ingredient to leave a kind of 'imprint' on the molecules of water used to dilute it – and this imprint is replicated from dilution to dilution. Critics deride this idea. Despite the best efforts of supporters to demonstrate the validity of this imprinting, it has to be accepted that if homeopathy does indeed work, its mechanism remains obscure. A few practitioners are keen to prove that homeopathy is effective when tested by standards similar to those which are routine in orthodox medicine. A couple of scientifically conducted trials appear to have shown that homeopathy does indeed work. But this number is pretty small in comparison with the tens of thousands of such experimental tests which have been carried out on conventional drugs. As with most alternative medicine, the scientific jury is still unconvinced.

Like most practitioners of alternative medicine, the homeopath will spend much longer than a conventional doctor finding out about each patient. And while conventional medicine is apt to prescribe according to the patient's symptoms, homeopathy prescribes according to the patient him or herself. So although two people may have the same disorder, they won't necessarily be judged suitable for the same treatments. And the treatment which is selected will be adjusted or even changed completely according to how the patient responds to what he has already been given.

Manipulation

There are at least half a dozen forms of manipulative therapy, but the most widely practised in Britain is osteopathy. During the patient's first visit the osteopath will take a full history, and carry out a detailed examination of the patient's posture, standing and sitting, and the way that he or she moves. The examination may also involve orthodox medical techniques such as blood pressure measurement, X-rays, and urine analysis. What the osteopath is looking for are any misalignments or other abnormalities of the body's muscles and bones. Having identified any such disturbances, one or more of a number of techniques can be used to correct them. Massage of specific muscles or parts of muscles which are deemed to be tense or otherwise stressed in some way is a common feature of treatment. Osteopaths also have a deep interest in the movement of the body's joint; they aim to free any stiffness and allow a fuller range of movements by, for example, stretching shortened ligaments. Of course, the technique which most of us associate with osteopathy – especially those who have experienced it first hand – is the high velocity thrust. These are sudden movements which cause the joint under manipulation to crack – not always totally without pain.

It takes little imagination to accept that manipulation

might have something to offer in dealing with joint or muscular disorders – and indeed it is aching backs and the like which prompt most of those who visit osteopaths to do so. But how could such techniques help – in this instance – an irritable bowel? There are certain theoretical explanations to account for the link; but most osteopaths nowadays are less concerned with the rather doubtful theory originally invoked by the founder of their discipline, and more with practical results. Although they accept that relatively few people come to consult them about non-musculo-skeletal conditions, they claim that many also experience unexpected benefits as far as other disorders are concerned.

Herbalism

Of all the alternative therapists, this is the one with which the sceptic has the the least trouble coming to terms. Herbalism is after all the forerunner of today's orthodox drug treatments. Indeed, some of the pharmaceutical industry's products are no more than refinements or derivatives of the basic ingredients of the herbalist's own medicine chest. The advent of pharmacology as a science, and the rise of the pharmaceutical industry, nearly put paid to herbalism. But it survived and today, like other forms of alternative medicine, is on the increase.

The use of plants to treat illness is at least as old as recorded history, and presumably a good deal older. Even today, every primitive or peasant society maintains a stock of its own remedies. In many parts of the Third World these are the only medicines which people can afford. As with many other non-scientific or pre-scientific systems of medicine, the attempt to heal the body by brews, potions, and tinctures cannot be divorced from the relationship of the healer and healed to each other and to the world in which they live. In other words, the personal elements of herbalism have always been, and to a degree remain, a valued ingredient. It is this, as much as the nature of the medicines themselves, which sets herbalism apart from the drug-prescribing of the GP.

There are many different forms of herbalism, each with its own views, procedures and remedies; many herbalists use one or several other alternative techniques of diagnosis and treatment in parallel with their own medicines. They tend not to diagnose illness in the way that a doctor might. They are less concerned with identifying discrete diseases, and more interested in the way the body is functioning or failing to do so. Having defined what they perceive to be the nature of the failure, they then prescribe whatever they believe will best restore that function to normal. Herbal remedies are designed to provoke the body into healing itself; to adjust its physiological and chemical processes when these have, for whatever reason, got out of kilter; and to encourage it to eliminate toxins and other waste materials. Herbalists are also concerned with the causes of whatever they perceive to be the source of the imbalance, and will encourage patients to change the way they live if this is felt to be responsible for whatever has prompted the patients to seek help.

The remedies themselves are usually made by drying plant roots, leaves or flowers as appropriate, chopping them finely, and then leaving them to soak in a solvent of some kind – usually a mixture of alcohol and water. This infusion is then filtered and pressed to obtain a tincture suitable for use as a medicine. When the pharmacologist finds that a particular herbal medicine really does have a specific effect on the body, his inclination is to purify and extract the active ingredient from among the variety of different substances which are apt to be found in most such remedies. The thinking here is that only a pure and standardized preparation can be counted upon to give consistent results. The herbalist, on the other hand, makes a positive virtue of not attempting to separate out the active ingredient. He will argue that in combination with other materials present in the plant extract, the active principle is sometimes more effective, or less likely to cause side effects, or both.

Healing

If herbalism is the technique with which orthodox medicine has the least trouble coming to terms, healing might seem to lie at the opposite end of the spectrum. It could also be argued that this is the purest form of alternative medicine: one which places no reliance on instruments and potions which, sceptics would argue, have no effect anyway. Healing relies solely on the innate capacity of one human being to heal another.

In so far as prayer is a form of healing, it is a feature of many of the world's religions. But the term is usually taken to mean something more specific than the vicar's brief mention during Sunday morning prayers of Mrs Jones who's been feeling a bit poorly of late. The practice of healers varies considerably. A few are full-time professionals, but most charge no fee. Some conduct their healing at a distance, without ever having met their subject. But it is more common to conduct the healing with the subject there in front of them.

The healer will normally want to find out a little about the person, and what's wrong with him or her. During the healing itself the subject will normally be seated with eyes closed, and asked to relax. The healer may then place his or her hands over or on the affected part – hence the phrase 'laying on of hands'. Any notion that this is a deeply private experience which can only be conducted in dim light and a quiet room is dispelled by the sight of a healing display at one of the increasingly popular exhibitions of alternative medicine. I remember one in

London which featured half a dozen healers, all wearing white coats and each concentrating on the person seated in front of them. The cluster of healers, undistracted by the attention and the noise around them, carried out their healing with no more fuss than might be expected of someone demonstrating a kitchen gadget at the Ideal Home Exhibition.

What is actually happening during the healing session? The answer you'll get will depend on who you ask. Most healers regard themselves as a channel for the transfer of healing energy into the person they are trying to help. Some see that energy as coming from God; others believe it comes from within themselves. To the sceptical scientist, healing is a particularly powerful instance of the placebo effect. The subject responds to the healer's belief in his or her powers with an equal acceptance of those powers. What follows is a self-fulfilling prophecy in which the patient's condition improves because this is what the patient believes will happen. The mechanism of the placebo effect is obscure, but all sorts of plausible explanations can be put forward to account for the power of belief to, for example, boost the effectiveness of the immune system.

To say that alternative medicine will cure nothing is as silly as saying it will cure everything. But the relationship between alternative and conventional medicine remains ill-defined and uncomfortable. Until recently it was a professional offence for a doctor to refer patients to unorthodox practitioners, or indeed to have anything to do with them. The hypocrisy of this stance can be appreciated when you recall that some doctors themselves made use of certain of the forbidden fruits, especially osteopathy, against which they publicly warned their patients. Attitudes have softened a great deal in recent years. An increasing minority of doctors now make an effort to learn certain alternative techniques. While many others continue to doubt that their patients will benefit by unorthodox remedies, few would nowadays actively try to prevent their patients from seeking such help – provided it doesn't conflict with whatever advice or treatment they themselves are offering.

12 Other Functional Disorders

Still glides the Stream, and shall
  for ever glide;
The Form remains, the Function never
  dies.

William Wordsworth, 'The River Duddon'

The main features of the irritable bowel syndrome are pain in the abdomen together with constipation and/or diarrhoea. As if getting to grips with the IBS itself isn't problem enough, the picture becomes even more confusing in that each of these symptoms can occur in isolation. When this happens the treatment is chosen, of course, to match the symptom in question. But that's not all; functional disorders of the gut – those in which doctors have not yet found any kind of physical abnormality – aren't limited to these particular symptoms; singly or in combination. None of these further disorders is as common as the irritable bowel syndrome – but each one is every bit as perplexing. This chapter will look at four of them, the intention being to illustrate something of the full range of unpleasantness to which the human gut is heir.

Non-ulcer dyspepsia

Dyspepsia is the smart term for indigestion: in other words, pain and discomfort of the lower chest or upper abdomen, usually following meals, and originating in the higher reaches of the gastrointestinal tract. It may be accompanied by belching, fullness, nausea and bloating; the pain may be better at night, or become worse. Abdominal pain is regularly experienced by people suffering from ulcers of the stomach or duodenum; indeed, the word dyspepsia is sometimes equated with such ulcers. The term 'non-ulcer dyspepsia' makes it clear that it is possible to have bad indigestion in the absence of an ulcer, or indeed of any other sign of physical disease. Would-be connoisseurs of indigestion might like to know that an upsurge of interest in the topic has led enthusiastic researchers to recognize no less than five types of dyspepsia. (Just for the record the other four are essential dyspepsia, ulcer-like dyspepsia, flatulent dyspepsia and the rather grandiose 'epigastric distress syndrome'. Some doctors favour still more subdivisions.) Non-ulcer dyspepsia is very common, and there is a distinct overlap in symptoms between it and the irritable bowel syndrome.

The cause of non-ulcer dyspepsia is still a matter of speculation – but it may well be another consequence of abnormal gut motility. One line of evidence came originally from the study of a patient who had complained for years of feeling that his stomach was bloated. Normally when one eats a meal, the lower part of the stomach will begin to contract powerfully. In the man with dyspepsia these contractions were largely absent. And while the liquid contents of his stomach were released into the next stretch of the gut – the duodenum – at more or less the expected time, the emptying of the solid contents of his stomach was much delayed. Other studies of other patients have confirmed the existence of this unusual pattern of activity. But this relative underactivity wouldn't by itself explain why solid food is retained; it seems likely that there is also a failure of the muscles surrounding the exit from the stomach to relax at the appropriate moment and so allow free passage of the stomach contents.

There are several ways in which abnormal muscle activity could cause the symptoms of non-ulcer dyspepsia. Spasm of the muscles themselves could give rise to the pain. Alternatively the discomfort could be provoked by the contents of the duodenum flooding back into the stomach, or by the stomach contents being forced back into the gullet; or the whole thing might be to do with prolonged retention of food in the stomach. As if to confound such speculation, some patients with dyspepsia seem to have perfectly normal motility; it is indeed difficult to prove that abnormalities of motility are responsible for the symptoms of non-ulcer dyspepsia.

As with the irritable bowel syndrome, all sorts of explanations for the abnormality have been mooted: possible failures of the nervous and hormonal systems have generated much speculation; other researchers have talked of the patients' personalities and neuroses. Stress too has had a good innings; there is evidence that this can delay the rate at which the stomach discharges its contents into the duodenum. In one series of experiments, volunteers agreed to swallow a tube which could then be used to measure the rate of stomach emptying. All were required to immerse one hand in a tub of water; but while half the subjects did so in water at room temperature, the remainder had to put their hands into ice cold water. This simple form of stress had a marked delaying effect on the rate at which material left the stomach. If stress affects all of us in this way, it is not difficult to see how some people who might be more conscious of stress, or who might respond more strongly to it, could then develop the symptoms of non-ulcer dyspepsia. But this is only one theory among many.

Drugs which stimulate the muscles of the stomach to greater activity do, as you might predict, offer some relief to patients with this form of dyspepsia. But many go on taking antacids or drugs designed to suppress their production of acid.

Burbulence

Burbulence is the technical and rather splendid term for those symptoms arising from an excess of gas in the stomach. Its most obvious consequences – belching and flatulence – are not the most physically uncomfortable of its effects, but socially they are the most distressing. There have been times – and there still are places – where a noisy release of gas – a belch – is not only acceptable, but positively welcomed as indicating approval of whatever food has been provided. In Britain this is not so . . . but do not be too swift to condemn transgressors. Some belching is less a failure of good manners than an irrepressible response to physiological forces beyond human control. Escape of excess gas through the lower orifice is nowhere interpreted as complimentary – though it may, of course, be equally unstoppable.

Less disconcerting for others, though much more so for the sufferers themselves, are the bloating and abdominal pain which may result from too much intestinal gas. This is sometimes attributable to an inability to belch, and so relieve the pressure. But what is this gas, and from where does it come?

The gut produces around two litres of gas every day, and at any one moment contains up to a couple of hundred millilitres. (There is, in medicine, virtually nothing which someone, sometime, somewhere hasn't chosen to study and measure.) The gas itself comprises a mixture of carbon dioxide, nitrogen, oxygen and hydrogen. It may also contain methane and hydrogen sulphide – components which help to create the characteristic odour. The hydrogen, carbon dioxide and methane are largely the result of bacterial action within the large bowel. The reason that bean-eating is so often an anti-social act is that beans contain certain carbohydrate molecules which can't be digested by the enzymes present in the small bowel. As a consequence these carbohydrates aren't absorbed – and pass on through to the large bowel. Here the resident bacteria feast with enthusiasm on their unexpected treat – with gaseous results. (It is worth recalling, incidentally, that humans are rank amateurs in this business of gas production. According to one set of calculations, the cattle population of America produce enough methane to account for 8 per cent of the household needs of the US human population.)

The other source of gas in the gut is swallowed air. While flatulence is primarily gas produced by bacteria, it is this swallowed air which accounts for most of the volume of a belch. All of us swallow a certain amount of air during normal eating; but some people take in more than their fair share. During normal breathing, air is sucked from the back of the throat, down the windpipe and into the lungs. To prevent food and drink entering the airways, their entrance is protected by a flap of tissue called the epiglottis. If one contrives to breathe in while keeping the epiglottis closed, some air will pass not into the windpipe but the oesophagus. Most of this will escape during the next outward breath – but some may reach the stomach. Many people who swallow air are completely unaware of what they are doing. Some people do it during their sleep, and quite a few of us do it when we're nervous.

Returning briefly to intestinal gas: the presence of hydrogen and methane renders this inflammable, or even explosive. One surprising circumstance in which this has been known to prove hazardous is during surgery. When small blood vessels are cut during an operation it has long been customary to seal them using a technique known as electrocautery. This involves passing an electric current through the bleeding points using the forceps or whatever other instruments have been used to locate them. The local tissue heats up and, in the case of a blood vessel, is sealed. Sometimes this process induces a small spark. If the surgeon has just opened up a bowel containing inflammable gas, he may inadvertently ignite it. The only person who doesn't suffer a degree of shock at such moments is the anaesthetised patient; but it is his bowel which bears the brunt of the physical injuries resulting from the explosion. This is not a theoretical hazard, incidentally; it really has happened. The safety-conscious surgeon can minimize the risks to all concerned by, among other manoeuvres, cleansing the bowel before an operation is commenced.

Remedies for burbulence are many and various. Avoidance of high risk food and drink – from carbonated beverages to baked beans – is the most obvious way of dealing with the problem. As some flatulence is caused by dietary fibre on which the bacteria of the large bowel may feed, cutting out materials such as bran may help. But in view of the benefits of fibre, this is not without disadvantages. One way to determine which food or foods are responsible for the problem is to adopt the approach used to find out if a particular food is causing IBS symptoms. In other words, switch to the simplest possible diet, then reintroduce regular foods one at a time and see if the gas problem re-erupts.

Drug therapy for the problem takes various forms. Antacids may help; so may powdered charcoal, kaolin and chalk – none of which are particularly appetizing. Materials called 'defoaming agents', originally developed to overcome bloating in cattle, encourage small bubbles of gas to coalesce to form larger ones which, in theory, escape more easily from the liquid trapping them in the gut. Cinnamon, ginger and peppermint are all believed on the basis of minimal evidence to reduce flatulence. The history of materials used for this purpose – they're known collectively as 'carminatives' – goes back several thousand years. If you like old-fashioned remedies, these are for you.

Proctalgia fugax

This little known and even less understood disorder is an acute, unexpected, infrequent, and sometimes quite excruciating pain in the region of the rectum. Although more women than men tend to suffer from it, anyone at any age can fall victim. Some attacks may follow a visit to the lavatory which has involved an undue amount of straining; others appear to be brought on by sexual activity; others still by fatigue. There seem to be no hard and fast rules. The pain itself builds up swiftly, lasts from a few seconds to several minutes, and has been described by one sufferer as not unlike having a wedge shot into the anus. It tends to leave the sufferer shocked and, given the relative brevity of the discomfort, with a surprisingly intense feeling of exhaustion. The source of the pain almost certainly lies in one of the several muscles which surround the point at which the rectum meets the anus, and are responsible for maintaining continence and allowing defecation. The muscle presumably goes into a spasm – though it is difficult to be sure because any one episode will be long gone by the time a doctor has had a chance to examine the patient.

Relatively few people go to the doctor on account of proctalgia fugax, and the complaint may be far more common than is generally realized. Between a tenth and fifth of the population seem to experience it at one time or another. The tiny minority who do seek a medical opinion will, as usual, find that all the doctor can do is eliminate everything which proctalgia fugax is not: pelvic disease in women, for example; or an inflamed prostate in men.

Treatments are idiosyncratic. Some find relief in cold, others in heat, still more in pressure. Adopting a doubled-up posture may help; 'doubled-up in pain' here takes on a literal meaning. The precise ways of applying these remedies depend only on the ingenuity of the sufferer and the circumstances, public or private, under which the attack has taken place. All sorts of drugs have been tried, but without any evidence of benefit. The most valuable help which the doctor can provide is reassurance that proctalgia fugax is nothing to worry about. Patients may take some convincing on this point; it is after all rather difficult to believe that something so acutely painful signifies nothing.

Globus

Ascending now from the lower to the upper end of the gastrointestinal tract, we find something which as many as half of us experience from time to time: a lump in the throat. A disproportionate number of the people who have this sensation – or at any rate report it to their doctors – are women. Doctors being largely male, could this be one reason why the disorder is often known as globus hystericus?

The 'lump' causes no pain and usually seems to lie just beyond and below the back of the throat: in other words at the upper end of the oesophagus. Some sufferers are aware of it all the time; others only when they eat or drink. In some people the sensation of having a lump may result from tension in one of the muscles at the back of the throat. Another theory has it that the sensation is a consequence of more general feelings of tension. Tense people, it's argued, swallow repeatedly. As they run out of saliva they become aware of greater swallowing difficulty – and so of the lump-in-the-throat sensation. If this notion is correct, anyone should be able to create the sensation by repeated swallowing. You can try it for yourself. More fanciful theories invoke suppressed emotion as the cause of the sensation. These ideas derive, as you might guess, from the universal experience that powerful emotion induces the lump sensation. These theories merit full marks for ingenuity; but probably less for validity.

Beyond explanation and reassurance, it is hardly surprising to learn that for globus there is . . . no treatment.

13 Living with the Irritable Bowel Syndrome

> The guts uphold the heart, not the heart the guts.
>
> Proverb

It was not my intention, in writing this book, to spell out some kind of ideal or 'correct' way of treating the irritable bowel syndrome. If, by now, you have formed the view that there is no such thing as an ideal remedy, you have the picture exactly. Indeed, if the IBS is not really one condition but several – at this stage indistinguishable from each other – then by definition there is no such thing as a single ideal treatment. As you may also have gathered, doctors differ widely among themselves about the true nature of the syndrome. To summarize the theories reviewed in this book, they include: lack of dietary fibre; food intolerance; an abnormality of the muscles of the gut; an abnormality of all smooth muscle in the body; a hormone disturbance; a failure of the normal relationship between the enteric and central nervous systems; stress; psychiatric disorders; hyperventilation; and learned illness behaviour. That's quite a selection to choose from – and there may be others which I've missed. It is not really surprising that doctors are divided on how best to treat the condition.

If there is a 'typical' treatment, it is probably a recommendation to eat more fibre, and/or take a bulking agent, along perhaps with a drug. The more unusual treatments such as hypnotherapy or food intolerance investigations will be offered only if you happen to be dealt with by a gastroenterologist who takes a particular interest in such matters. Seeking treatment for the IBS can prove to be extremely dispiriting – and Professor David Wingate of the London Hospital provides an all-too-exact summary of how and why the relationship between doctor and patient can spiral into mutual distrust and irritation.

The patient and the doctor: what can go wrong

Let's see it first from the patient's point of view. Imagine someone who has suffered for years from the IBS, who has been visiting the doctor on and off during much of that time, and whose symptoms still haven't improved much. That person may have lost count of the number of times he has seen the doctor. He will have had all kinds of tests and examinations that probably haven't revealed anything; collected several diagnoses which even the doctors making them don't seem sure about; listened to a series of explanations which strike him as frankly unlikely if not downright evasive; and finally been prescribed several treatments which have all failed to deal with the problem. These events are all too likely to implant a series of suspicions in his mind. Why so many consultations? Perhaps the doctor doesn't understand. And all those tests which turned out negative may mean that the doctor just wasn't ordering the right ones. Maybe the doctor doesn't really know what is wrong ... or, worse, he does know but he's hiding something. Of course, he *must* know what's the matter or he wouldn't be prescribing treatment. But the treatment isn't working; so maybe the doctor's incompetent ...

Suspicion, of course, breeds fear. Maybe the doctors aren't really interested in me. Maybe I've developed a tumour which they can't find. Or maybe they have found it, and they're afraid to tell me. Perhaps it's too late anyway ...

This is how Professor David Wingate believes it can look from the patient's point of view.

WHAT THE PATIENT EXPERIENCES
○ multiple investigations
○ negative investigations
○ dubious diagnoses
○ evasive explanations
○ ineffective therapy

WHAT THE PATIENT THINKS
○ multiple investigations
  The doctor doesn't understand
○ negative investigations
  The doctor has ordered the wrong tests
○ dubious diagnoses
  The doctor doesn't know
○ evasive explanations
  The doctor is hiding something
○ ineffective therapy
  The doctor is incompetent

WHAT THE PATIENT FEARS

○ multiple investigations
  The doctor isn't interested

○ negative investigations
  They can't find the tumour

○ dubious diagnoses
  They don't know what's wrong

○ evasive explanations
  They're afraid to tell me

○ ineffective therapy
  It's too late!

From the doctor's point of view things look quite different. He too, of course, is equally conscious that all the consultations and investigations have turned up no sign of organic disease. The treatment he has prescribed has achieved nothing, and he is left having to confront an extremely unhappy patient. From Professor Wingate's experience, the doctor's thoughts are likely to be running along the following lines. First, because of the repeated consultations, the doctor may come to feel that the patient is wasting his time. Indeed, the absence of any sign of organic disease may prompt him to wonder if his patient really is ill anyway. The negative investigations will likely as not reinforce that suspicion – as will the poor response to treatment. And what conclusion can be drawn about a patient who is manifestly unhappy and imagining all kinds of symptoms? Of course: depression.

This is how Professer Wingate suggests it can look from the doctor's point of view.

THE EXPERIENCE OF THE DOCTOR
- ○ repeated consultations
- ○ no signs of organic disease
- ○ negative investigations
- ○ poor response to therapy
- ○ an unhappy patient

WHAT THE DOCTOR THINKS
- ○ repeated consultations
  The patient is wasting my time
- ○ no signs of organic disease
  The patient seems to be perfectly well
- ○ negative investigations
  There's nothing wrong, just as I thought
- ○ poor response to therapy
  The symptoms must be imaginary
- ○ an unhappy patient
  Aha! Obviously this is depression

This outline of what happens is deeply depressing; but it is all too easy to see how, in view of the uncertainties about the IBS, the relationship between doctor and patient can spiral into mutual antagonism. Even if the doctor explains everything there is to be explained, and the patient makes an effort to listen, take things in, and not expect miracles, misunderstandings can still arise. As neither doctors nor patients are likely to be perfect, some degree of misunderstanding is virtually inevitable. Professor Wingate himself tries to minimize it by taking a positive approach to his patients, by trying to avoid using treatments which aren't very likely to work, by explaining as much as he can about what he is doing and why, and above all by emphasizing that while the outlook may not be encouraging, the IBS is neither life threatening, nor a harbinger of worse disease yet to come.

Parallels with ME

Irritable bowel syndrome patients face much the same kind of problem as that confronting people with ME: myalgic encephalomyelitis, or the post-viral fatigue syndrome. Although only relatively recently recognized (at least by most people) as a genuine disorder, ME has succeeded in acquiring much more publicity than IBS. This in turn has not only created a wider awareness of the existence of ME, but even persuaded both doctors and lay people to take it a little more seriously than they might once have been inclined to do, and even to offer some genuine sympathy. Indeed, the parallel with ME is rather instructive.

Like the IBS, myalgic encephalomyelitis comprises a collection of different symptoms: a syndrome, in other words. These symptoms affect the central nervous system and the muscles, and different individuals will experience them in different combinations and with different degrees of severity. Its main features are muscle pain and fatigue, loss of memory and concentration, and continual feelings of tiredness and malaise. In addition there are a whole collection of further symptoms which some ME patients may suffer. These include depression, cold feet and hands, a sore throat, tender glands, headaches, dizzy spells, palpitations, breathlessness, sleep disturbances and – most intriguingly – a number of the symptoms of the irritable bowel syndrome. (So far as I know, nobody has yet suggested that ME and the IBS have a similar cause – though given the number of theories put forward to account for the two conditions, it can only be a matter of time.) The symptoms of ME may appear suddenly or slowly, they fluctuate from day to day or month to month without apparent pattern, there is no evidence of physical abnormality in the patient's body, and the problem may persist for years.

The response of doctors to ME has been enormously varied. At first many refused to believe that the condition even existed. Their reactions were consequently predictable: some patients were dismissed as hypochondriacs; others as neurotic worriers about their health; and some were simply accused of malingering. (A few doctors, incidentally, still take this view.) Attempts to understand the illness got off to a bad start when, in 1955, one of the earliest well-documented outbreaks affected many of the staff at London's Royal Free Hospital. Indeed ME is still sometimes referred to as 'Royal Free Disease'. Extensive investigation showed absolutely nothing amiss with the Royal Free Staff who went down with the illness. This led to the suggestion that they had been suffering from an hysterical illness: in other words, one which originates in the mind and which, moreover, can sometimes sweep through a group of people as more and more of them become convinced that they too are suffering from whatever it is. Epidemics of hysteria, in which people become oddly suggestible and develop the symptoms shown by others around them, do seem to occur, though not frequently. So this kind of hysterical illness is a real disorder, albeit a psychiatric one. However, the suggestion that Royal Free Disease might be an hysterical illness prompted an almighty row. And it wasn't entirely a straightforward desire to know the truth which prompted the commotion.

The strength of feeling suggests that many of the doctors and nurses involved took great exception to the notion that they might have been suffering from a psychiatric disorder. Coming from professions which take great pains to assure the rest of us that there's no disgrace or stigma in being given a psychiatric diagnosis this was, to say the least, unfortunate. Happily this phase of the argument about ME is largely over, and there is general agreement that it is most likely to be a condition provoked by a virus that lingers in the body long after it should have been eliminated, or which sets up some kind of abnormal immune response which continues to trouble the patient even when the guilty virus has long since departed.

Malingering

There are a number of parallels between ME and the irritable bowel syndrome. Neither has yet been associated with any physical abnormality in the body, and both are very difficult to diagnose except by eliminating everything that they are not. Both are characterized by a handful of core symptoms and a variety of others from which patients may or may not suffer, and which are variable and unpredictable. And while both conditions are acutely real to sufferers, both are poorly defined.

A great many people who have suffered from ME have found themselves accused of malingering. For obvious reasons this charge is very difficult to rebut; and it has to be conceded that anyone who *is* set on malingering will find in either ME or the IBS a very satisfactory excuse. There really seems no way around this problem: genuine patients in both groups have little option but to learn to live with a certain level of suspicion. If you are accused of faking your symptoms, the temptation must be to respond abusively if not physically. On the whole this temptation is best resisted. A reasoned attempt to explain what you know about the syndrome is more likely to serve you well in the long run.

Practicalities

The irritable bowel syndrome is a chronic complaint; suffering just one or two bouts of pain in the stomach coupled with constipation or diarrhoea should not be taken as tantamount to an automatic diagnosis of the IBS. If the problem recurs, go to your doctor – not specifically to find out if the IBS is the true cause of the problem, but because misbehaving guts should be investigated anyway. Occasional diarrhoea may not be greatly troublesome, but it can indicate that something organic is wrong; and why endure a troublesome symptom when there's always the possibility that something simple may stop it. You may be one of those people who doesn't like or even distrusts conventional medicine, and prefers to find advice and treatment from an alternative practitioner. If that person isn't him or herself medically qualified, it really is worth going to a conventional GP – and being referred if necessary to a hospital specialist – before you seek any other therapy. You may not like what conventional medicine has to offer, but no one is going to oblige you to follow whatever advice or treatment you are given. It is at least worthwhile seeing and talking to a conventional doctor. They are the people best placed to find out if what you have got is worth worrying about. A lot of hospital consultants have got their favourite stories about patients who arrived in their clinics almost at death's door because a fringe practitioner had been treating them for something relatively trivial, not realizing that the apparently minor symptoms which had prompted the patient's visit were in fact the warning signs of something potentially lethal. This may not happen often – and almost certainly not as often as some doctors would have you believe. But preventable mistakes shouldn't happen at all.

Assuming that you do decide to follow the doctor's advice, give it a fair try. If the treatment recommended is even marginally troublesome it is tempting to cut corners and follow instructions only half-heartedly. By all means abandon the treatment if you have tried it conscientiously for a couple of months and seen no improvement. Given that an irritable bowel never killed anyone, that is a sensible decision. Likewise if the improvement is so slight as to leave the treatment more troublesome than the illness, again abandon it. But don't give up on the doctors altogether. Make another appointment if one isn't already booked, pass on the bad news about the failure of whatever has been prescribed, and ask if the doctor has any other ideas which might be worth considering. If he hasn't, and your inclinations are anyway to give alternative medicine a try, this is probably the time at which to do so. Your GP may be sympathetic, and may even be prepared to help your choice. Or he may not – in which case you are on your own in the matter of selection.

If you know any other patients with the IBS, talk to them about their condition. Most people with chronic disorders devise ways of coping which simply wouldn't occur to any professional, and which may never cross your mind either. As yet in Britain there doesn't seem to be a patient self-help group working in this area. Why this is so I'm not sure as there are patient groups for even the most rare and obscure disorders – and while the IBS may be obscure, it is certainly not rare. The burgeoning of the patient self-help movement in recent years is testament to the benefits which sufferers derive from these groups. At its most basic they provide the comfort of knowing that you are not alone: that other people too have the illness and thus share the misery. Their newsletters and meetings provide an opportunity for swapping information of the kind already mentioned. And some of the groups flourish to the extent that they start raising funds with which to support research into their illness. In some cases research initiated by a patient support group has successfully brought a hitherto neglected disorder out of the cold, and on to the research agenda.

Stress

The argument about stress and the part it plays in provoking the irritable bowel syndrome is unresolved. But that is no reason for neglecting it. Whatever you may think about the importance or otherwise of stress, it is unlikely that trying to minimize its effects on your life is going to do anything but good. Stress reduction is notably free of side effects. So how best to set about it? The first step is to spend some time thinking about how you live and how you behave at work and at home, and towards friends and relatives, bosses and subordinates. Think how you relax – if you do at all – and how you spend your spare time. Whole books are written on this topic, and all I'll do here is indicate the sort of questions you might be asking yourself.

- ○ Am I doing the right job? Is it the one which best suits my personality?

- ○ Am I too busy? Or not busy enough?

- ○ Should I be living in a town, or would I be better off in the country? But if I couldn't change job, would commuting be even worse?

- ○ Am I sacrificing my home life to my work?

- ○ Do I spend long enough with my friends?

- ○ Am I placing too many demands on myself?

- ○ Are other people making too many unreasonable demands of me?

- ○ Could I make life easier for myself by reorganizing it in some way?

The list of questions of this kind is virtually endless; but only you can know which are the right ones to ask – and what are, for you, the answers.

The general principles to be followed in responding to questions like these have become know as 'stress management'. One of its basic tenets is that you should periodically examine all your goals and priorities, and ask yourself if they are the right ones. If what you are aiming to achieve is unrealistic or unlikely to give you a sense of fulfilment when you have achieved it, there really isn't much sense in striving for it. But you do have to know yourself well before you can make decisions like this. A minority of people experience the greatest frustration not through failing to achieve an ambitious goal, but because they have no goal for which to strive. It is easy to confuse a busy and hectic life with a stressful one. Working long hard hours isn't necessarily stressful, if that is what you genuinely find satisfying. Again, you have to know yourself if you are to make the right changes.

Exercise

Regular exercise can help. It has similar effects on many of the body's systems to those induced by stress – but with very different consequences. The rise in heart rate, blood pressure and adrenaline output which accompany exercise are directed to some purpose, and do not merely have to be dissipated in pointless rage and frustration. The psychological value of exercise is also beneficial. This is difficult to account for, but may have something to do with natural chemicals called endorphins which seem to be generated during intense exercise. The emotional uplift which comes with certain forms of intense exercise (the 'runner's high') are thought by some scientists to be the consequence of an increased output of endorphins.

Meditation, yoga and autogenics

Relaxation and biofeedback have already been mentioned. They were described in previous chapters in the context of efforts to use them directly in tackling the irritable bowel syndrome. But as ways of learning to relax they might also have an indirect value. Other techniques which can promote relaxation are meditation, yoga and autogenic training. The object of meditation is to induce a state of peace and quiet inside your head. There are many methods; some are derived from, or are part of, a formal religious tradition – Zen Buddhism, for example. Others are wholly secular. But most of them have certain features in common, especially the requirement that the meditator directs all his concentration on to a single word, or picture, or fundamental activity such as breathing. All conscious thought should be allowed to drain away. Studies of the electrical activity of the brains of people meditating reveal marked changes: notably an increase in the activity within the right hemisphere of the brain. This is the half which is more concerned with artistic as opposed to rational thought patterns. People who have mastered the technique of meditation say that they feel revitalized, but at the same time more calm.

Yoga comes in many forms, some of which emphasize physical health and others of which are little different in nature and intent from meditation. But despite these variations in emphasis, all are concerned with the relationship of body and mind, the aim being to achieve a state of harmony between the two. In practice this is achieved by a series of poses and exercises together with careful control over breathing. Many of the positions adopted by people doing yoga look appallingly uncomfortable; but with practice they are not. Of course, the novice doesn't start out by wrapping his legs around his neck in the way that advanced students can manage with relative ease. Many of the poses and exercises are very simple, and the body becomes increasingly supple with use.

Yoga was in existence at least 5,000 years ago; autogenic training, devised in the twenties, has a less impressive pedigree. It comprises bits and pieces of several techniques including yoga, hypnosis and various other relaxation techniques. The idea behind it is to concentrate on a particular part of the body, and then try to influence the state of feeling or performance of that part. This is usually achieved by silent repetition of a phrase such as 'My legs feel warm and heavy'. By moving around from part to part – limbs, trunk, neck, head and so on – the whole body can be induced to relax. With practice, the repetition of the key phrase or phrases at difficult or tense moments should induce a rapid relaxation. You could describe autogenic training as a way of learning how to turn off the 'fight or flight' response when it's inappropriate – as it usually is when summoned up by the kinds of stress which most of us face in the twentieth century. The person who has managed to cast off the stress response should then find himself better able to concentrate on whatever it is he is trying to do.

There are nowadays so many competing methods of relaxation that it is virtually impossible to recommend one as against another. Moreover a great deal depends on personal preference: someone who can't get on with yoga may take immediately to autogenics, and vice versa. There is no way to find out which, if any, will suit you except by giving each one a try.

If the theory of the type A/type B personality is correct, it is the competing, aggressive type A who is most likely to need and to benefit from stress management.

Type As may not be able to change their personality type; but they should be able to mitigate its worst effects.

Personally speaking

I do not suffer from the irritable bowel syndrome; but I am plagued quite regularly by mild stomach rumbling – or borborygmus as I must try remembering to call it. This condition could hardly be described as having more than minor nuisance value. But even this trivial complaint has given me an insight into the distress caused by more severe functional disorders of the gut.

My rumbling is fairly predictable and usually confined to the morning hours: seldom before 9.30 a.m., and not often later than 11.30 a.m. No doubt its appearance is connected with my preference for a light breakfast: coffee and one slice of toast. As often as not I hardly notice the rumbling – and would probably never have given it much thought had it not been that, as a broadcaster, I spend a fair proportion of my time sitting in quiet studios in front of sensitive microphones. The background noise of a stomach rumbling can come through with startling clarity. When interviewing someone it is virtually impossible to ask a serious question, or listen to a serious answer, if both parties are well aware of a gurgling sound in the background. On many occasions I have had to call a halt to the interview or the discussion, and put the question again or ask the interviewee to repeat the answer. But there are times when, although I feel a stirring in the stomach which I know is about to become a rumble, I am reluctant to interrupt the flow of what may be a difficult argument or train of thought. In such circumstances I go through a ritual of largely useless ploys in an effort to suppress the rumble. Sometimes I tense the muscles of my abdomen in the hope of forcing the unruly stomach to behave itself. Alternatively I slide my chair forward so that the edge of the desk in front of me is pressed firmly against my belly. Sometimes I slide the chair backwards from the microphone in the hope of putting my gut beyond the audible range. None of these manoeuvres works; only desperation drives me to them. Lord knows what other people in the studio make of these antics. On one humiliating occasion – when proceedings had already been stopped three times on account of rumbles audible to the producer listening in the control cubicle – I abandoned my studio guest, ran three floors to buy a sausage roll, then gobbled it down before her bemused gaze. The interview continued – without my rumbles, but with my contributions sounding rather more breathless than before.

Only once has my stomach rumble been recorded under circumstances in which a repeat performance was impossible; the tape just had to be abandoned. Moreover, by remembering to eat even a modest snack a few minutes before going into the studio, I can usually forestall problems. As you may appreciate, in the sum total of difficulties which face human beings, mine are pretty modest. And most people I work with regard the whole thing as a joke. I am probably the only one who doesn't always find it funny.

The point of going into so much detail about such a small thing is that the nature of my work makes it, to me, a nuisance and an embarrassment. And if I can be discomforted by something as trivial as an uncontrollable stomach rumble, it stands to reason that someone with a fullblown irritable bowel will find it proportionately more troublesome. So to those reading this book who themselves suffer from the IBS I can only say that while I don't suffer from your disease, I do have a faint glimmering of your predicament.

Final thoughts

To round things off, let me once more summarize what seems to me a sensible approach to take if you do develop the core symptoms of the irritable bowel syndrome: that is, abdominal pain plus diarrhoea and/or constipation. Once you've decided that it isn't going to clear up of its own accord, visit your doctor and ask his advice. If whatever treatment he offers doesn't seem to work, go back and tell him. He may want to try something else, or he may refer you for a hospital appointment. Once again, follow the same approach: take the advice and treatment that's offered, and don't be afraid to seek further help if the problem is getting no better. If the doctors you've seen appear to be running out of ideas, press them to refer you for a less orthodox treatment – and don't be deterred if they show some reluctance. If they can't – or won't – refer you for hypnosis or whatever (and remember that they may quite genuinely not be able to on the NHS), use the addresses in the back of this book to help you find a qualified practitioner. There's nothing to prevent you trying whatever self-help remedies you hear of at any stage of this progression – *provided* that what you choose to do doesn't interfere with any other treatment which is being prescribed. Your doctor will be able to advise you.

The irritable bowel syndrome won't necessarily last for ever. Some people do find that orthodox medicine provides a rapid solution. Others are troubled for a couple of years or even a decade, and then their IBS suddenly vanishes of its own accord. Always remember that the irritable bowel syndrome is one of those disorders in which treatment is most likely to be successful when you *don't* leave all responsibility for a cure to the doctor.

What you do for yourself may be as valuable as anything which medicine can do for you.

Useful Addresses

These bodies will supply a list of approved practitioners in their field of interest. They appreciate a stamped and self-addressed envelope.

Association for Applied Hypnosis
33/39 Abbey Park Road
Grimsby
South Humberside DN32 0HS

British Association for Counselling
37a Sheep Street
Rugby
Warwickshire CV21 3BX

British Homeopathic Association
27a Devonshire Street
London W1N 1RJ

British Hypnotherapy Association
1 Wythburn Place
London W1

British Society of Medical and Dental Hypnosis
PO Box 6
42 Links Road
Ashtead
Surrey KT21 2HT

General Council and Register of Consultant Herbalists
Marlborough House
Swanpool
Falmouth
Cornwall TR11 4HW

National Council of Psychotherapists and Hypnotherapy
  Register
1 Clovelly Road
London W5

National Federation of Spiritual Healers
Old Manor Farm Studio
Church Street
Sunbury-on-Thames
Middlesex TW16 6RG

National Institute of Medical Herbalists
41 Hatherley Road
Winchester SO22 6SR

*More general enquiries about alternative medicine should
be directed to:*

The Institute for Complementary Medicine
21 Portland Place
London W1N 2AF

Glossary

acetylcholine A chemical produced by nerve endings to instruct muscle fibres to contract.

adrenaline A hormone with many actions on the body – including preparation for 'fight or flight'.

allergy Sensitivity to specific materials which is mediated by the body's immune defence system.

anti-cholinergic A drug which disrupts the acetylcholine message system.

anti-spasmodic A drug designed to relax muscles.

anus The orifice through which the rectum discharges faeces.

anxiolytic A minor tranquillizer; a drug used to reduce anxiety.

autonomic nervous system The part of the nervous system which is responsible for regulating bodily processes such as blood pressure and digestion which are outside conscious control.

benzodiazepine Drugs of Valium type; used to treat anxiety.

biofeedback A technique in which subjects use special

instruments which allow them to become aware of physiological events such as brain activity and blood pressure.

borborygmus A technical term for stomach rumbling.

bran The outer layers of each grain of wheat, removed during milling if the object is to prepare white flour.

bulking agent Material designed to increase the weight and volume of stools.

burbulence Symptoms caused by excess gas in the stomach.

carbon dioxide Gas produced by respiration, and exhaled.

cellulose Material of which plant cell walls are made. A component of dietary fibre.

central nervous system The brain and spinal cord.

cholecystokinin A hormone which, among other things stimulates the gallbladder.

colon The large intestine excluding the rectum.

colonoscopy A technique for examining the interior of the colon. Flexible viewing tubes now allow doctors to examine most of its length.

controlled trial A method of assessment in which a drug or other treatment is compared with some other treatment, or with a dummy (placebo) pill or procedure.

diaphragm The layer of muscular tissue which separates the chest cavity from the abdominal cavity.

diverticular disease Pain and disturbed bowel habit associated with pouches which form at weak points on the wall of the colon.

duodenum The section of the intestine into which partially digested food moves on leaving the stomach.

dyspepsia Indigestion; usually applied to pain or discomfort in the abdomen or lower chest following meals.

endorphins Natural chemicals which are thought to modulate sensitivity to pain.

enteric nervous system The complex of nerve cells found throughout the wall of the gut.

enzyme A natural substance which speeds the rate at which certain chemical processes take place within the body.

fibre The indigestible components of our diet.

flora The pattern of bacterial types found in a particular location in the body, such as the gut.

food intolerance Any adverse reaction to a food.

functional disorder Any illness in which there is no discernible physical or chemical abnormality which might be causing the problem.

gastroenterologist A doctor specializing in diseases of the gut.

globus The sensation of having a lump in the throat.

homeopathy The system of medicine based on the principle of 'Like cures like'.

hydrogen breath test A method of finding out how long food takes to reach the large bowel.

hyperventilation Overbreathing; breathing too deeply or rapidly, with adverse consequences.

ispaghula Dried plant seeds used as bulking agent.

lactase An enzyme which breaks down lactose sugar into smaller molecules.

lactose A type of sugar found only in milk.

lignin A component of dietary fibre.

ME Myalgic encephalomyelitis: ill-understood fatigue which betrays no physical evidence of its existence, but produces profound weakness and malaise in sufferers. May be caused by an unusual response to a virus infection of some kind.

migrating motor complex The term for a sequence of muscular contractions which stir food in the small intestine, and move it along.

oesophagus The gullet; the tube which carries food from the mouth to the stomach.

organic disorder A disorder which can be traced to a specific chemical or structural abnormality or failure in the body.

osteopathy Form of treatment based on manipulation of muscles and joints.

parasympathetic system One of the two branches of the autonomic nervous system.

pectin A type of dietary fibre.

peptic ulcer An ulcer which appears in the lining of the gut or stomach.

peristalsis Waves of contraction in the gut muscles which keep food moving through the intestine.

placebo A dummy pill, treatment or procedure.

placebo effect A form of self-healing in which the effect of a drug or other treatment results not from the treatment itself, but from the patient's expectations of benefiting by it.

proctalgia fugax A sudden and brief pain in the region of the anus.

psychosomatic symptoms Bodily symptoms provoked by the influence of the mind.

psychotherapy Any kind of talking treatment for psychological or psychiatric disorders.

psychotropic drug Any kind of drug which acts on mood or emotions.

ptyalin An enzyme found in saliva.

pyloric sphincter The muscular valve guarding the exit from the stomach.

receptor The specialized area of a cell's surface which responds to chemical messages such as hormones.

rectum The final section of the gut, and the part where faeces are stored prior to being expelled through the anus.

roughage An older term for dietary fibre.

segmentation movements Muscular contractions of the gut.

sigmoidoscope A viewing tube used to examine the interior of the lower reaches of the large bowel.

smooth muscle Muscle found in many of the body's hollow organs, including the gut. Produces long, slow contractions which are not generally under voluntary control.

spastic colon An older name for the irritable bowel syndrome; also used to describe one set of IBS symptoms.

sphincter A muscular valve which closes off a tube in the body.

sympathetic system One of the two branches of the autonomic nervous system.

syndrome A collection of symptoms which, when they

occur together, are regarded as constituting a distinct illness.

transit time The time required for the passage of food from mouth to anus, or through some other specified length of the gastrointestinal tract.

typeA/typeB A distinction made between two personality types which shape people's response to, among other things, stress.

vagus nerve   A nerve which carries signals to and from the brain and various of the body's organs.

villus A tiny inward projection of the lining of the gut; large numbers of them serve to increase its surface area.

Index

NOTE: Irritable Bowel Syndrome is abbreviated to IBS; numbers in italics refer to diagram.

A Full List of Cedar Books

While every effort is made to keep prices low, it is sometimes necessary to increase prices at short notice. Mandarin Paperbacks reserves the right to show new retail prices on covers which may differ from those previously advertised in the text or elsewhere.

The prices shown below were correct at the time of going to press.

☐ 434 11163 5	**When Am I Going to be Happy?:**	Dr Penelope Russianoff	£4.99
	How to Break the Emotional Bad Habits		
	That Make you Miserable		
☐ 434 11156 2	**Living with M.E.: A Self-help Guide**	Dr Charles Shepherd	£4.99
☐ 434 11126 0	**How to Increase Your Sales to Industry**	Alfred Tack	£4.99
☐ 434 11111 2	**How to Increase Your Sales by Telephone**	Alfred Tack	£4.99
☐ 434 11106 6	**How to Overcome Nervous Tension and**		
	Speak Well in Public	Alfred Tack	£4.99
☐ 434 11110 4	**How to Succeed as a Sales Manager**	Alfred Tack	£4.99
☐ 434 11125 2	**How to Succeed in Selling**	Alfred Tack	£4.99
☐ 437 95156 1	**Marketing: The Sales Manager's Role**	Alfred Tack	£3.50
☐ 434 11132 5	**1000 Ways to Increase Your Sales**	Alfred Tack	£4.99
☐ 434 11105 8	**The Courage to Grieve: Creative Living,**		
	Recovery and Growth, Through Grief	Judith Tatelbaum	£4.99
☐ 434 11122 8	**Seeds of Greatness: the ten best-kept**		
	secrets of total success	Denis Waitley	£3.95
☐ 434 98172 9	**Letters of a Businessman to His Son:**	G. Kingsley Ward	£4.99
	'The Extraordinary Book that has Changed		
	a Million Business Lives'		

All these books are available at your bookshop or newsagent, or can be ordered direct from the publisher. Just tick the titles you want and fill in the form below.

Mandarin Paperbacks, Cash Sales Department, PO Box 11, Falmouth, Cornwall TR10 9EN.

Please send cheque or postal order, no currency, for purchase price quoted and allow the following for postage and packing:

UK	80p for the first book, 20p for each additional book ordered to a maximum charge of £2.00.
BFPO	80p for the first book, 20p for each additional book.
Overseas including Eire	£1.50 for the first book, £1.00 for the second and 30p for each additional book thereafter.

NAME (Block letters) ....

ADDRESS ....

....

....